Studien zur Mustererkennung

herausgegeben von:

Prof. Dr.-Ing. Heinrich Niemann
Prof. Dr.-Ing. Elmar Nöth

Bibliografische Information der Deutschen Nationalbibliothek

Die Deutsche Nationalbibliothek verzeichnet diese Publikation in der
Deutschen Nationalbibliografie; detaillierte bibliografische Daten sind
im Internet über http://dnb.d-nb.de abrufbar.

ISBN 978-3-8325-3726-5
ISSN 1617-0695

Logos Verlag Berlin GmbH
Comeniushof
Gubener Str. 47
10243 Berlin
Tel.: +49 030 42 85 10 90
Fax: +49 030 42 85 10 92
INTERNET: http://www.logos-verlag.de

3-D Imaging of the Heart Chambers with C-arm CT

3D-Bildgebung der Herzkammern mit C-Bogen-CT

Der Technischen Fakultät
der Friedrich-Alexander-Universität
Erlangen-Nürnberg

zur

Erlangung des Doktorgrades Dr.-Ing.

vorgelegt von

Kerstin Müller

aus

Nürnberg, Deutschland

Als Dissertation genehmigt
von der Technischen Fakultät
der Friedrich-Alexander-Universität Erlangen-Nürnberg

Tag der mündlichen Prüfung:	09. Mai 2014
Vorsitzende des Promotionsorgans:	Prof. Dr.-Ing. habil M. Merklein
Gutachter:	Prof. Dr.-Ing. J. Hornegger
	Assoc. Prof. R. Fahrig, Ph.D

Abstract

Nowadays, angiography is the gold standard for the visualization of the morphology of the cardiac vasculature and cardiac chambers in the interventional suite. Up to now, high resolution 2-D X-ray images are acquired with a C-arm system in standard views and the diagnosis of the cardiologist is based on the observations in the planar X-ray images. No dynamic analysis of the cardiac chambers can be performed in 3-D. In the last years, cardiac imaging in 3-D using a C-arm system becomes of more and more interest in the interventional catheter laboratory. Furthermore, the analysis of the 3-D motion would provide valuable information with respect to functional cardiac imaging. However, cardiac motion is a challenging problem in 3-D imaging, which leads to severe imaging artifacts in the 3-D image. Therefore, the main research goal of this thesis was the visualization and extraction of dynamic and functional parameters of the cardiac chambers in 3-D using an interventional angiographic C-arm system.

In this thesis, two different approaches for cardiac chamber motion-compensated reconstruction have been developed and evaluated. The first technique addresses the visualization of the left ventricle. Therefore, a whole framework for left ventricular tomographic reconstruction and wall motion analysis has been developed. Dynamic surface models are generated from the 2-D X-ray images acquired during a short scan of a C-arm scanner using the 2-D bloodpool information. The acquisition time is about 5 s and the patients have normal sinus rhythm. Due to the acquisition time of about 5 s of the C-arm, no valuable retrospective ECG-gated reconstructions are possible. The dynamic surface LV model comprises a sparse motion vector field on the surface, which can be used for functional wall motion analysis. Furthermore, applying various interpolation schemes, dense motion vector fields can be generated for a tomographic motion-compensated reconstruction. In this thesis, linear interpolation methods and spline-based methods have been compared. The combination of the wall motion analysis and the motion-compensated reconstruction is of great value to the diagnostic of pathological regions in cardiac interventions.

The second motion-compensated reconstruction approach uses volume-based motion estimation algorithms for the reconstruction of two - left atrium and left ventricle - to four heart chambers. A longer C-arm acquisition and contrast protocol allows for the generation of initial images at various heart phases. However, the initial image quality is not sufficient for motion estimation. Therefore, different pre-processing techniques, e.g., bilateral filtering or iterative reconstruction techniques, to improve the image quality were tested in combination with different motion estimation techniques.

Overall, the results of this thesis highly demonstrate the feasibility of dynamic and functional cardiac chamber imaging using data from an interventional angiographic C-arm system for clinical applications.

Kurzfassung

Heutzutage ist die fluoroskopische Angiographie das meist eingesetzte Verfahren zur Darstellung von Koronargefäßen und Herzkammern. Jedoch ist die Herzkatheteruntersuchung mit Hilfe eines angiographischen C-Bogens beschränkt auf die Analyse von 2D Röntgenbilder. Allerdings würde eine funktionale dreidimensionale Untersuchung des Herzens wichtige zusätzliche Information direkt im Katheterlabor bereitstellen. Basierend auf 2D Röntgenbildern, die während einer Rotation eines C-Bogen Systems aufgenommen wurden, können 3D Bilder des Körpers mit Hilfe von Rekonstruktionsalgorithmen berechnet werden. Allerdings stellt sich die 3D Darstellung des bewegten Herzens als sehr schwierig dar. Hinsichtlich der längeren Aufnahmezeit von mehreren Sekunden, verursacht die Herzbewegung Bildartefakte in der tomographischen 3D Rekonstruktion. Demzufolge war es das Hauptziel dieser Arbeit, Algorithmen und Möglichkeiten zu entwickeln, welche die 3D Darstellung des Herzens mit einem C-Bogen System erlauben und mittels verschiedener Verfahren funktionale Parameter des Herzens zu extrahieren.

In dieser Arbeit wurden zwei unterschiedliche Ansätze zur bewegungskompensierten Rekonstruktion von Herzkammern entwickelt und ausgewertet. Die erste Methode beschäftigt sich mit der Darstellung des linken Ventrikels. Hierfür wurde eine umfassende Anwendung zur bewegunskompensierten 3D Darstellung des linken Ventrikels und zu dessen Wandbewegungsanalyse entwickelt. Während der 5 s Aufnahme hat der Patient einen normalen Sinusrhythmus. Aufgrund der Aufnahmedauer können keine EKG-basierten Rekonstruktionen erfolgen. Daher wurde ein oberflächenbasiertes Verfahren entwickelt. Hierzu wird das 2D Blutvolumen in den Projektionsbildern segmentiert und unter Zuhilfenahme dieser segmentierten Daten werden dann dynamische Oberflächenmodelle generiert. Diese Modelle erlauben es die Bewegung an der Oberfläche zu bestimmen und diese für die Bewegungsanalyse zu nutzen. Für eine tomographische bewegungskompensierte Rekonstruktion werden jedoch dichte Bewegungsfelder benötigt. Diese dichten Bewegungsfelder können mittels verschiedenster Interpolationstechniken generiert werden, zum Beispiel mit linearen oder spline-basierten Methoden. Die Kombination aus funktioneller und bewegungskompensierter, tomographischer Darstellung hat einen hohen Wert für die Diagnose von pathologischen Regionen während der kardiologischen Untersuchung.

Der zweite Ansatz arbeitet mit volumenbasierten Techniken zur Herzbewegungsschätzung. Für diese Anwendung wird nicht nur das linke Ventrikel, sondern auch das linke Atrium beziehungsweise alle Herzkammern dargestellt. Hierfür wird ein Aufnahmeprotokoll mit längerer Aufnahmezeit benötigt. Die Aufnahmetechnik erlaubt es 3D Bilder des Herzens in verschiedenen Bewegungszuständen zu visualisieren. Allerdings ist die Qualität dieser initialen Bilder nicht ausreichend für einen klinischen Einsatz. Deswegen wurden verschiedene Vorverarbeitungsschritte, zum Beispiel ein bilaterales Filter oder iterative Rekonstruktionsverfahren, zur Bildqualitätsverbesserung in Kombination mit 3D Bewegungsschätzung und -kompensation untersucht.

Zusammenfassend zeigen die Ergebnisse der Arbeit, dass erste Ansätze für die Anwendung von dynamischer und funktioneller Herzbildgebung mit einem angiographischen C-Bogen im klinischen Umfeld möglich sind.

Acknowledgement

It always seems impossible until its done. - Nelson Mandela

Managing a comprehensive project like this PhD project cannot be done without being surrounded by creative, eager and dedicated people. The whole project has only been possible due to the help and support of many people. I would like to express my wholehearted appreciation to anybody who has contributed to this thesis, lightened up some of my working days and made me enjoy my work. In particular, I would like to thank

Prof. Dr.-Ing. Joachim Hornegger for giving me the opportunity to work on such an interesting research topic over the years, even before my PhD. I really appreciate his excellent and professional support - beyond this thesis, and during my work at the Pattern Recognition Lab. Thank you for giving me the chance to work in such an inspiring and kind working atmosphere.

Dr. Günter Lauritsch, there are no words which could express how thankful I am that you have been my Siemens advisor for the last years. Thank you for the uncountable time, patience, and for numerous discussions about the project, my papers and many more things. Thank you for your continuous support, you always made me believe that I can actually get all the work done. I also really enjoyed our conversations beyond research and I will definitely miss all the hiking activities during our travels.

Dr.-Ing. Andreas Maier for his 24h support. All our discussions have been very encouraging and helped me a lot to publish all the papers during the course of this thesis and to actually finish the thesis. Thank you for telling me that everything will be fine in the end, and I should not worry to much about it!

Assoc. Prof. Rebecca Fahrig, Ph.D. for countless proof readings of all my papers. Furthermore, I am very thankful for every discussion about my project and its future directions when I was visiting Stanford. Also big thanks to you and your team, Teri, Erin, Cameron, Wendy and many more for their help to discuss the acquisition protocols and for the actual acquisition of the data.

I also would like to thank Dr. med. Carl Schultz at the Thoraxcenter, Erasmus MC, The Netherlands (now at the School of Medicine and Pharmacology, Royal Perth Hospital Unit, Perth, Australia) and Priv.-Doz. Dr. med. Harald Rittger at the Universitätsklinikum Erlangen, Germany for providing the clinical data for the left ventricle analysis. I also would like to say thank you to Prof. Dr. Hein Heidbüchel and Dr. Stijn De Buck at the University Hospital Gasthuisberg, University of Leuven, Belgium to provide the experimental porcine datasets. Furthermore, I would like to thank Dr. med. Bernd Abt and Dr. med. Henning Köhler at the Herz- und Kreislaufzentrum Rotenburg a. d. Fulda, Germany for providing the clinical data. It was a pleasure for me to work with all of you.

Furthermore, I would like to thank all my colleagues at the LME and at the Siemens AG which made the last three and a half years unforgettable. If somebody would ask me if I would do the same project again, I would definitely say: "Yes!". I also thank my student Steffen Fiedler, who did an excellent job and hopefully comes back to the lab for his master thesis. I could thank so many more people at the lab for the discussions during coffee breaks, MAGs or any other occasion, you all contribute to the familiar working atmosphere at the lab which I really enjoyed working in.

Thanks to Eva Eibenberger and Jana Hutter, I think we did a pretty good job for medical engineering. I enjoyed working with you! Hope to meet you from time to time, either in Germany, USA or UK!

I also owe a big *Thank you* to my "reconstruction twin" Chris Schwemmer. I cannot imagine how the three years would have been without our discussions and your helpful comments when I was struggling with a problem. Working together was fruitful and I would say that we had quite a bit of fun while working, traveling and cooking (also thanks to Christoph Forman!).

Thank you also goes to Christopher Rohkohl for his "emergency hotline", he was always willing to help if I encountered problems with the reconstruction framework. I definitely loved the virtual coding sessions!

Special thanks to my "Thesis Review Committee": Christopher Rohkohl, Günter Lauritsch, Andreas Maier and Alexander Brost, all provided me with valuable feedback and comments and made the impossible possible in a very short amount of time.

Last but not least, I thank my parents and my boyfriend Matthias for their mental support, patience and encouragement during the last years. Thank you for your rare complaints when I sometimes spent more time working than I probably should have.

Erlangen, May 19th 2014   Kerstin Müller

Contents

Chapter 1 Introduction   **1**
1.1 Heart Anatomy and Cardiac Cycle   2
    1.1.1 Heart Anatomy   2
    1.1.2 The Cardiac Cycle and the Actions of the Valves.   3
1.2 Clinical Relevance of 3-D Cardiac Imaging   4
    1.2.1 Cardiac Ultrasound (US)   5
    1.2.2 Computed Tomography (CT)   6
    1.2.3 Magnetic Resonance Imaging (MRI)   6
    1.2.4 Nuclear Imaging   7
    1.2.5 Angiography & C-arm CT   7
    1.2.6 Discussion   8
1.3 C-arm CT for 3-D Rotational Angiography.   8
1.4 Scientific Contribution to the Progress of Research 10
1.5 Structure of the Thesis 12

Chapter 2 State-of-the-Art in 3-D Cardiac Imaging   **15**
2.1 General Notation of Reconstruction Algorithms 16
2.2 Static Image Reconstruction 16
    2.2.1 Analytical Cone-beam Image Reconstruction. 17
    2.2.2 Iterative Image Reconstruction 18
    2.2.3 Geometric Image Reconstruction 23
2.3 From Static to Dynamic Image Reconstruction. 23
    2.3.1 Single Sweep ECG-Gated Image Reconstruction 24
    2.3.2 Multiple Sweep ECG-Gated Image Reconstruction 25
2.4 Motion Estimation Techniques 26
    2.4.1 3-D/3-D Image Registration 26
    2.4.2 2-D/3-D Image Registration 27
    2.4.3 2-D/2-D Image Registration 28
2.5 Motion-Compensated Image Reconstruction. 28
    2.5.1 Motion Compensation in 2-D Projection Space 28
    2.5.2 Motion Compensation in 3-D Image Space. 29
2.6 Joint Motion Estimation and Compensation. 30
2.7 Difference to Cardiac Vasculature Image Reconstruction 30
2.8 Challenges in Clinical Applications 32
2.9 Summary and Conclusions 32

Chapter 3 Surface-based Motion Estimation, Reconstruction & Analysis   **33**
3.1 Motivation and Clinical Applications 34
3.2 Acquisition and Contrast Protocol 35

3.3 Motion Estimation and Compensation via Surface Model. 35
   3.3.1 Initial Surface Mesh Generation. 36
   3.3.2 2-D Bloodpool Segmentation 36
   3.3.3 Heart Phase Identification 36
   3.3.4 Dynamic Surface Model Generation. 38
   3.3.5 Different Motion Interpolation Techniques 38
   3.3.6 Cutting 41
   3.3.7 Motion-Compensated Reconstruction. 41
   3.3.8 Complexity Analysis. 42
   3.3.9 Implementation Details and Parameter Setting 42
3.4 Ventricle Motion Analysis 43
   3.4.1 Left Ventricle Representation 43
   3.4.2 Motion Analysis 44
3.5 Evaluation and Results 46
   3.5.1 Motion Estimation and Reconstruction 46
   3.5.2 Wall Motion Analysis. 59
3.6 Challenges. 72
3.7 Summary and Conclusions 73

Chapter 4   Volume-based Motion Estimation and Reconstruction   75
4.1 Motivation and Clinical Applications 76
4.2 Acquisition and Contrast Protocol 77
4.3 Motion Estimation and Compensation via Registration 77
   4.3.1 Initial 3-D Volume Generation. 77
   4.3.2 3-D/(3+N)-D Objective Function & Optimization Strategy 85
   4.3.3 Final Image Reconstruction 92
4.4 Complexity Analysis 93
   4.4.1 Initial 3-D Volume Generation. 93
   4.4.2 3-D/(3+N)-D Registration. 94
   4.4.3 Motion-compensated Reconstruction. 95
4.5 Implementation Details and Parameter Setting. 95
   4.5.1 Initial 3-D Volume Generation. 95
   4.5.2 3-D/(3+N)-D Registration. 96
4.6 Evaluation and Results 99
   4.6.1 Datasets 99
   4.6.2 Quantitative Evaluation Methods of 3-D Reconstruction Quality 102
   4.6.3 Edge Response Function 103
   4.6.4 Experimental Results 104
4.7 First Clinical Patient Data 119
4.8 Challenges. 122
4.9 Summary and Conclusions 122

Chapter 5   Summary and Outlook   125
5.1 Summary. 125
5.2 Outlook 128

List of Abbreviations and Symbols   129

List of Figures   137

List of Tables   139

List of Algorithms   141

Bibliography   143

CHAPTER 1

Introduction

1.1 Heart Anatomy and Cardiac Cycle 2

1.2 Clinical Relevance of 3-D Cardiac Imaging 4

1.3 C-arm CT for 3-D Rotational Angiography 8

1.4 Scientific Contribution to the Progress of Research 10

1.5 Structure of the Thesis 12

The European Society of Cardiology published the fourth edition of the European cardiovascular disease statistics in 2012 [Euro 12]. They stated that diseases of the heart and blood circulatory system are the main cause of death in Europe, accounting for over 4 million deaths each year. It is also the main cause of death for people younger than 65 years in Europe. The potential risk of a patient to suffer from any kind of coronary heart disease can be determined by the so called "Framingham Risk Score" [Wils 98]. The Framingham risk score uses categorical variables, e.g. gender, age, blood pressure, and total cholesterol, to predict coronary heart disease risk in patients without indicating symptoms for heart diseases. If a patient indicates any type of cardiac disease, several examinations need to be performed, e.g. a stress electrocardiogram or stress echocardiogram. If the patient is diagnosed with a heart disease, the patient will undergo an interventional coronary procedure. Nowadays, coronary angiography is the gold standard for the visualization of the morphology of the cardiac vasculature and chambers [Krak 04]. Up to now, high resolution 2 D X-ray images are acquired with a C-arm CT system in fixed views and the diagnosis of the cardiologist is based on the observations in the planar X-ray images. From these, no dynamic analysis of the cardiac chambers can be performed in 3-D. In the last years, cardiac imaging in 3-D gains more and more interest in the interventional catheter laboratory. Cardiac motion is a challenging problem in 3-D imaging, which leads to severe imaging artifacts in the 3-D image. The analysis of the motion provides valuable information with respect to functional cardiac imaging. Therefore, the main research goal of this thesis is the visualization and extraction of dynamic and functional parameters of the cardiac chambers in 3-D using an interventional angiographic C-arm system.

In this chapter, a short introduction to the heart anatomy and the cardiac cycle is given in Section 1.1. Furthermore, the importance and clinical relevance of cardiac imaging, especially interventional cardiac imaging with a C-arm CT system is presented in Sections 1.2 and 1.3. This chapter ends with a summary of the achieved

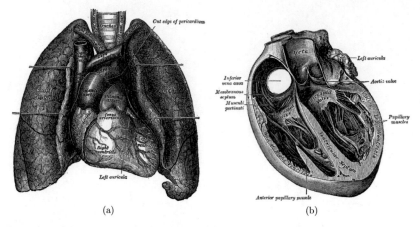

(a)   (b)

Figure 1.1: Schemes of the heart anatomy. (a) Front view of the heart and the lungs. (b) Scheme of the human heart which shows the two ventricles and the septum. Images taken from [Gray 00].

scientific contributions of this thesis to the progress of research and with an overview of the individual thesis chapters in Sections 1.4 and 1.5.

1.1 Heart Anatomy and Cardiac Cycle

In this section, the heart anatomy and cardiac cycle are briefly described. The description is completely based on the work of Henry Gray in the book „Anatomy of the Human Body" (1821 to 1865). Only relevant anatomic details are given below - for further details the reader is referred to the public domain online book of Henry Gray [Gray 00].

1.1.1 Heart Anatomy

An adult human heart is a hollow muscular organ and is located between the lungs in the middle of the mediastinal cavity, see Figure 1.1a. It is placed behind the sternum and located generally farther into the left than into the right half of the thoracic cavity. The heart measures about 12 cm in length, 8 to 9 cm in width and 6 cm in depth. The weight varies for males between 280 to 340 grams and for women from 230 to 280 grams. Both, size and geometry of the heart change with increasing age [Kitz 90]. Also variations can be observed between athletes and others in the normal general population [Maro 06]. In general, the heart consists of four chambers. It is divided into a right and left half by the septal wall or septum. Both halves are further divided into two cavities, the atrium and the ventricle. The right atrium is usually larger than the left, but has a thinner wall measuring about 2 mm. The left atrial wall measures about 3 mm in thickness. The right and left ventricle are roughly of the

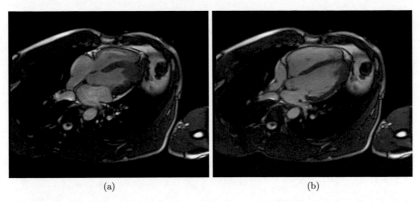

(a)   (b)

Figure 1.2: 2-D cine acquisition with a Magnetom Prisma MR scanner (Siemens AG, Health-care Sector, Erlangen, Germany) of the heart chambers at systole (a) and end-diastole (b) in an axial view.

same size, but the walls of the left ventricle are about three times as thick as those of the right one, as it needs to pump the blood through the whole body. A scheme of the human heart is given in Figure 1.1b. The heart itself consists of muscular fibers and fibrous rings. It is covered by the visceral layer of the epicardium and lined by the endocardium. In between these two membrane layers is the muscular wall, the myocardium. The endocardium is a thin, smooth membrane which forms the inner surface of the heart. The endocardium consists of connective tissue and elastic fibers, and is attached to the muscle by loose elastic tissue which contains blood vessels and nerves. A more detailed overview of the heart anatomy can be found in the online book of Henry Gray [Gray 00] and in the human anatomy atlas of Frank H. Netter [Nett 08b].

1.1.2   The Cardiac Cycle and the Actions of the Valves

When the heart is contracting, the blood is pumped through the whole body via the arteries. Each wave of contraction or period of activity is triggered from the sinus-atrial node. Every contraction period (systole) is followed by a period of rest, denoted as diastole. The two periods form the cardiac cycle. Example MRI reconstructions of the heart in systole and end-systole are given in Figure 1.2. Each cardiac cycle consists of three phases: (1) a short contraction of both atria, called atrial systole, followed by a small pause, (2) a prolonged contraction of both ventricles, denoted as ventricular systole or systole and (3) a period of rest, where the whole heart is relaxing, named diastole. During (1), the blood is pumped from the left atrium into the left ventricle and from the right atrium into the right ventricle, respectively. Regurgitation into the veins is prevented by the contraction of their muscular layer. When the ventricles contract (2), the valve between left atrium and left ventricle (mitral valve, also called bicuspid valve) and the valve between right atrium and

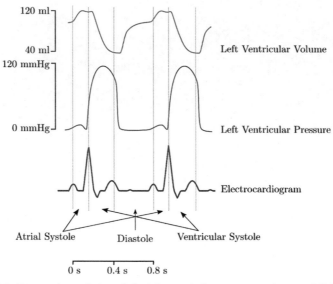

Figure 1.3: Temporal correlation of the left ventricular pressure, volume and ECG-signal over the heart cycle. Detailed scheme can be found in [Schr 09].

right ventricle (tricuspid valve) are closed to prevent the back flow of the blood into the atria. When the pressure inside the ventricles is high enough, the valves (aortic valve and pulmonary valve) into the aorta and pulmonary artery are opened and the blood is driven from the right ventricle into the pulmonary artery and from the left ventricle into the aorta. When the systole of the ventricle fades, the pressure inside the pulmonary artery and the aorta closes the valves to again prevent regurgitation. The valves remain shut until the next ventricular systole. During the period of rest (3), the tension of the mitral and tricuspid valve is relaxed, and blood flows from the veins into the atria and slightly also from the atria into the ventricles. The average duration of a cardiac cycle lasts about 0.8 s. It is divided into 0.4 s total systole (atrial: 0.1 s, ventricular: 0.3 s) and 0.4 s total diastole (atrial: 0.7 s, ventricular: 0.5 s). The temporal correlation between left ventricular pressure, volume and ECG-signal is illustrated in Figure 1.3. In Figure 1.4, the left ventricle, the aortic and the mitral valve are shown in a CT reconstruction at end-diastole.

1.2   Clinical Relevance of 3-D Cardiac Imaging

Death due to any kind of cardiac disease causes over 4 million deaths in Europe and 1.9 million deaths in the European Union. Cardiac vascular disease causes 47 % of all deaths in Europe and 40 % in the EU [Euro 12]. It was also the leading cause of death in the US in 2011 according to the Centers for Disease Control and Prevention

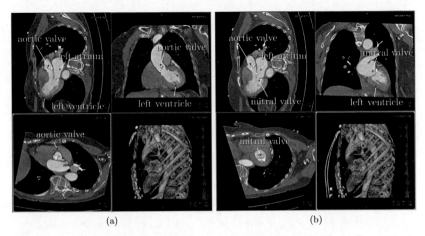

(a)   (b)

Figure 1.4: Somatom Definition Flash CT scanner (Siemens AG, Healthcare Sector, Forchheim, Germany) reconstruction at end-diastole, showing the mitral valve, aortic valve and the left ventricle in two different views (left/right) in multi-planar images and the volume rendering. The bright spots around the mitral valve and aortic valve are calcifications. The image data was provided by Dr. med. Abt and Dr. med. Köhler from the Herz- und Kreislaufzentrum Rotenburg a. d. Fulda, Germany.

of the National Center for Health Statistics (CDC/NCHS) [US D 12]. In addition to the therapeutic advances, the progress in cardiac imaging and diagnostics has lead to consistently declining death rates. The most common modalities for cardiac imaging are presented in the following paragraphs. The overview is based on Frangi et al. [Fran 01].

1.2.1   Cardiac Ultrasound (US)

Ultrasound (US), also called echocardiography, provides the ability to study the cardiac contraction behavior non-invasively via emitted ultrasound [Moyn 81]. Ultrasound is an easy tool for primary standard diagnosis of morphological or cardiac dysfunction. One limiting factor of this imaging modality is the attenuation of the ultrasound wave before it reaches the actual tissue of interest. Therefore, transesophageal echocardiography (TEE), transthoracic echocardiography (TTE), and intracardiac echocardiography (ICE) were developed in order to increase image quality for cardiac applications. Orienting the imaging slice in a 2-D scan can be challenging in an interventional setting using TTE [Jain 09]. TEE requires sedation of the patient, which may not be necessary for all cardiac interventional procedures. The ICE does not require the patient to undergo anesthesia and therefore, the use of ICE for mitral valve repair and electrophysiological procedures is growing [Hija 09]. Up to now, in contrast to TEE, ICE represents a purely intraprocedural guiding and navigation tool unsuitable for diagnostic purposes [Bart 13]. In recent years, three-dimensional echocardiography (3DE) allows quantitation of the heart in 3-D [Hung 07]. The 3DE is used to compute the ventricular volume over time and to perform wall motion analysis [Kape 05]. The 3DE images can also be registered and overlayed onto 2-D fluoroscopic images to enable soft tissue contrasting and functional imaging [Jain 09]. The parameter extracted from the 3DE exhibit some variances depending on the vendors analysis software [Sach 11]. Clinical studies were initiated to evaluate the deviations of the parameters among different software solutions [Mura 10, Wang 12].

1.2.2   Computed Tomography (CT)

Cardiac CT imaging is clinically important and can be used for diagnosis and risk analysis of coronary diseases. For example, for patients with an intermediate risk for coronary artery diseases, a so called coronary artery calcium (CAC) score can be assessed. In general, there exist two CT calcium scoring systems: the Agatston method and the "volume" score method [Budo 06, Qian 10, Erbe 07]. Both methods provide valuable information of atherosclerosis burden and for tracking changes over time in order to assess therapy efficacy [Budo 01, Hoff 03].

In CT systems, the hardware design limits the temporal resolution [Ache 06]. The acquisition is usually performed in a quiescent cardiac phase with less motion. However, the duration of the cardiac phase with small motion reduces with an increased heart rate. Image artifacts due to motion can occur in the reconstructions, especially in less advanced CT systems. Consequently, reconstruction algorithms that account for the motion need to be developed [Tagu 08, Schn 11, Rohk 13, Tang 12]. With new scanners, a temporal resolution of 75 ms can be achieved with a dual source CT system [Floh 08, Rohk 13]. In order to reduce radiation dose and to minimize the motion artifacts, minimum-dose scans are designed, which cover the whole heart during a single cardiac cycle, e.g., a high-pitch dual source CT spiral called "Flash spiral" or "Flash CT" [Ache 09].

In general, 4-D CT imaging is not performed for functional or dynamic analysis due to the high X-ray dose applied to the patient [Mang 05]. Furthermore, CT imaging can only be performed before or after the procedure for diagnosis, but not for interventional guidance or imaging.

1.2.3   Magnetic Resonance Imaging (MRI)

Cardiac MRI is a rapidly advancing technology for extracting functional and morphological information of the cardiac chambers and cardiac vasculature [Form 13]. Different acquisition sequences are used in order to acquire dynamic images of the heart. These images provide the ability to segment and to analyze the cardiac function [Matt 12, Ma 12]. Contrast enhanced MRI provides the possibility to show necrotic myocardial tissue. For the visualization of necrotic tissue, an additional scan after the administration of gadolinium-based contrast agent is performed about 10 min after the first non-contrast enhanced image aquisition [Mahr 08]. The necrotic tissue shows a higher concentration of contrast agent while the healthy tissue shows no contrast enhancement [Mahr 08].

In general, an MRI scan duration even with optimized scan sequences takes several minutes (6 min–10 min) [Form 13] and hence respiratory motion becomes a problem and needs to be taken into account [Nehr 01, Mank 02]. In general, MRI is used pre- or post-intervention for diagnosis, but in the recent years interventional MRI (iMRI) becomes of more and more interest [Kahn 12, Roth 11]. Interventional cardiac MRI is available in some clinics [Lede 06]. However, each device has to be designed specifically to work in a permanent magnetic field, leading to higher costs. Additionally, a challenging problem in MRI is imaging of patients with implantable devices, like permanent pacemakers. It is possible with special supervision and safety protocols, however, it is still dependent on the used MR system and the implanted device [Naza 13].

1.2.4   Nuclear Imaging

Myocardial perfusion scans play an important role in cardiac diagnostics. Positron emission tomography (PET) allows for perfusion and viability studies in order to find coronary artery diseases [Di C 07a, Schi 10]. Concerning the long acquisition time of a PET scan, respiratory and cardiac motion estimation and compensation techniques are required [Blum 10]. Another possibility is provided by the single positron emission tomography (SPECT) imaging. Despite that PET provides a higher sensitivity in the event counts, an improved image quality and shorter scans compared to SPECT, the workhorse in nuclear imaging is still SPECT imaging [Rahm 08]. This is due to the fact that a SPECT scan is cheaper than a PET examination [Kuwe 06, Di C 06], mostly due to the different tracer costs. Today, since PET and SPECT provide no valuable visualization of morphology, combined scans of SPECT/CT and PET/CT are performed to access the anatomic extent and the functional pathology in one scan [Di C 07b]. However, all presented modalities are for diagnostic use and do not provide interventional cardiac imaging.

1.2.5   Angiography & C-arm CT

Common cardiac procedures, e.g., pacemaker placement, valve repair and replacement or coronary vasculature assessment, are performed under interventional fluoroscopic X-ray imaging. These systems provide high resolution 2-D projection images during the intervention. Usually, contrast agent is administered intra-arterially or intra-venously to enhance vessels or corresponding tissue regions [Stro 09]. The C-arm system offers a high flexibility of imaging the patient from various views while providing accessibility to the patient during imaging. A combination of, e.g., a CT scan performed before the cardiac examination and the interventional 2-D acquired X-ray images from a C-arm system [Metz 13] can provide navigational assistance to the cardiologist. Additionally, angiographic C-arm systems provide volumetric computed tomography capabilities within the interventional suite [Fahr 97, Orth 09]. Therefore, the interest arises to use this system for 4-D (3-D+t) interventional imaging of the cardiac chambers.

1.2.6   Discussion

Most of the above presented modalities and techniques can only be applied before or after the intervention in order to provide quantitative and functional information about the heart and coronary vessels, e.g. CT or MR imaging. Therefore, the patient needs to be transferred from the interventional suite to another examination room for 3-D imaging and vice versa. Some modalities, e.g. MRI, are also limited to 2-D+t visualization, if imaging time plays an important role. TTE is also not feasible in an interventional setup, due to the positioning problem. TEE is able to overcome this problem, but requires sedation of the patient. ICE does not require anesthesia, however, it still provides only a limited field of view and a low image quality. Consequently, interventional 3-D+t imaging providing functional and morphological information can be further improved, which would then advance the outcome of cardiac diagnosis and procedures [De B 13a, Wiel 14].

1.3   C-arm CT for 3-D Rotational Angiography

The technical progress of the last decade allows for 3-D in-vivo imaging during clinical routine. One modality providing anatomical 3-D information of a patient is computed tomography (CT). However, these systems can only be applied pre- or post-interventionally, i.e. before or after the actual cardiac procedure. In between the acquisition and the intervention, the patient needs to be transferred from different examination rooms and patient beds. Therefore, a need for 3-D imaging directly in the catheter lab became of major interest in the mid-nineties [Roug 93, Sain 94, Fahr 97] and continued in the last years [Beck 09, Wall 09]. This interventional 3-D imaging can be performed with an angiographic C-arm CT system, already available in most catheter labs in order to perform 2-D fluoroscopic imaging. A C-arm CT system offers the possibility to acquire 2-D high-resolution X-ray images while the source-detector pair rotates around the patient. In order to be able to reconstruct a three-dimensional object from the acquired projection data, theoretical and technical difficulties need to be resolved [Orth 09, Wall 09]. For static objects enormous progress has been made over the last years [Zell 05, Stro 09, Stru 09].

In comparison to conventional CT imaging, the X-ray source and detector are mounted onto the flexible C-arm. Usually, the C-arm acquires projection data while performing a sweep around the patient, e.g., at least 200° degrees. In order to avoid artifacts caused by geometrical instabilities, the C-arm needs to be calibrated for each acquisition protocol to perform 3-D reconstruction. There exist also additional methods for online misalignment correction based on the reconstructed data, e.g., the image entropy is used as measure for misalignment [Wick 13]. Current state-of-the-art detectors in C-arm CT are flat-panel detectors to provide a homogenous image quality across the image, good 2-D soft tissue imaging and a dynamic range with 12 bits [Stro 09]. Table 1.1, shows a basic comparison to conventional CT systems.

Nowadays, most medical vendors offer C-arm CT solutions using C-arm systems equipped with a flat panel detector, called syngo DynaCT (Siemens AG, Healthcare Sector, Forchheim, Germany), XperCT (Philips Healthcare, Andover, MA), Innova CT (GE Healthcare, Chalfont St. Giles, UK), Infinix (Toshiba Corporation, Mi-

	CT	C-arm CT
Detector	multidetector ceramic	flat-panel
Number of detector rows	$\approx$ 100–320	$\approx$ 2000
Acquisition time (cardiac)	75 ms	5 s–15 s
Fluoroscopy	-	✓
Radiation/Dose	comparable	
Interventional	✗	✓
Spatial resolution	inferior	high
Contrast resolution	high	inferior
Flexibility	✗	✓
Scan field of view	$\approx$50 cm	$\approx$25 cm (large volume $\approx$47 cm)
Truncation artifact	moderate	severe
Scatter	moderate	high
Dynamic imaging	✗/✓	✓

Table 1.1: Difference between conventional CT and C-arm CT based on [Gupt 06, Kale 08, Ulzh 09, Stro 09].

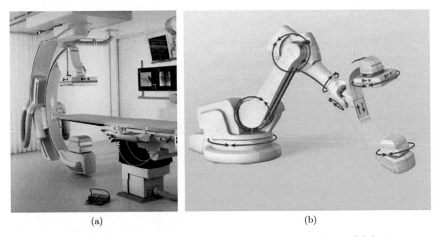

(a)   (b)

Figure 1.5: Example of C-arm systems: (a) Artis zee ceiling-mounted C-arm (b) Artis zeego (both Siemens AG, Healthcare Sector, Forchheim, Germany).

nato/Tokyo, Japan), and Trinias or Bransist (Shimadzu Medical Systems, Kyoto, Japan). Also companies in the small business sector, as Ziehm Imaging GmbH (Nürnberg, Germany) provides Ziehm Vision (FD) Vario 3D. Two variations of a C-arm system are given in Figure 1.5.

Several studies were published for different applications of C-arm CT, for example cardiac vasculature applications [Al A 08, Newe 09]. Furthermore, several research topics exploit the interventional C-arm CT data, e.g. transcatheter aortic valve implantation [John 10], 4-D digital subtraction angiography [Davi 13] and brain perfusion imaging [Manh 13]. However, due to the long acquisition time of the C-arm CT (several seconds), dynamic imaging is still an open and challenging problem [Rieb 09]. Therefore, the main research goal of this thesis is to develop and evaluate a concept for dynamic imaging of the heart chambers using a C-arm CT system. A detailed review of state-of-the-art algorithms for dynamic 3-D imaging is given in Chapter 2.

1.4   Scientific Contribution to the Progress of Research

In this section, the contributions of the thesis to the progress of research are shortly reviewed and the resulting scientific publications are listed below the individual topic.

Motion Estimation and Compensation

Motion estimation and compensation algorithms integrate the motion information in the reconstruction in order to use all acquired image data:

- A novel framework was developed for the computation of *dynamic surface meshes* of the left heart ventricle from a series of calibrated rotational 2-D X-ray images.

- For motion-compensated reconstruction, a dense motion vector field is required. Therefore, the sparse motion vector field, given by the dynamic surfaces meshes need to be extrapolated. Different *approaches to generate dense motion vector fields from the surface meshes* were evaluated with respect to the resulting reconstructed image accuracy and quality.

- Development of a complete new approach using a *3-D/4-D multiple heart phase registration* in order to estimate the cardiac motion between different heart phases. Here, a longer scan protocol of approximately 15 s is required.

- Development of a *motion estimation technique combined with a pre-processing pipeline utilizing 3-D/3-D registration* to provide motion-compensated reconstructions using a longer scan protocol of about 15 s.

The algorithmic contributions were presented at five international conferences [Chen 11, Mlle 12b, Mlle 12a, Chen 13c, Mlle 13d], parts of the work have also been published in two journal articles [Mlle 13c, Mlle 14b] and three patents have been filed [Chen 13a, Chen 13b, Mlle 13a] related to that topic.

Clinical Aspects

Novel technical development is the basis for the progress in medical imaging. In cooperation with our clinical partners, the following achievements were accomplished:

- *Design of a specific acquisition* and *contrast protocol* for imaging the left ventricle with a *5 s C-arm CT scan.*

- *Development of the first framework to perform quantitative analysis of left ventricular wall motion directly in the catheter lab using an interventional C-arm system.*

- All algorithms were tested on either *real clinical patient data* or on *comparable animal models.*

The acquisition protocol and the interventional wall motion analysis framework were published in one international conference publication [Mlle 12b] and two journal articles [Mlle 13c, Mlle 14c].

Phantom Creation for Research Community

The development and the evaluation of algorithms require commonly available datasets in the research community. In this thesis, three different simulated phantom datasets were created which are *publicly available:*

- *Design of a dynamic left ventricular heart phantom with contrasted blood in the aorta, myocardial wall and left ventricle.*

- A dense object, e.g., a *contrast-filled catheter can be placed inside the left heart ventricle* of the heart phantom. The same motion vector field as for the heart chambers is applied to the catheter. It allows evaluating the influence of streak artifacts due to dense objects on different motion estimation and compensation techniques. Two simulated datasets closely designed to real image data with a polychromatic spectrum similar to a clinical C-arm CT spectrum and monochromatic simulations are available.

- Left ventricular *phantom datasets modeling different pathological defects* were created in order to evaluate parameters for wall motion analysis. Akinetic and dyskinetic wall motion behavior was simulated to test the effect of the motion defect on the computed parameters.

The generated phantom data was presented on an international conference [Mlle 13b] and used in different publications [Mlle 13c, Mlle 13d, Maie 13, Mlle 14b, Mlle 14c, Mlle 14a].

In summary, the results of the thesis were presented on seven international conferences [Chen 11, Chen 13c, Mlle 12a, Mlle 12b, Mlle 13d, Mlle 13b, Mlle 14a] and three journal publications [Mlle 13c, Mlle 14b, Mlle 14c].

1.5 Structure of the Thesis

In this section, a chapter-wise overview of the thesis is given and acts as a direction through out the next chapters.

Chapter 2 State-of-the-Art in Cardiac C-arm CT

In the second chapter, a basic introduction to cardiac reconstruction algorithms using data acquired with a C-arm system is given. The necessary reconstruction notation is introduced as well as the geometry of the used C-arm device. In order to describe the dynamic reconstruction, first, the static reconstruction problem is explained in more detail. In clinical practice, an approximate analytical cone-beam reconstruction algorithm named FDK after the inventors Feldkamp, Davis and Kress [Feld 84] is used. In literature, also several iterative reconstruction techniques are presented, but up to now - to the best of the authors knowledge - no clinical C-arm scanner is applying an iterative reconstruction algorithm. For some applications, a tomographic reconstruction of the heart chambers is not required, but the geometry and morphology of the heart chambers might be of interest. Hence, geometric reconstruction type algorithms are shortly described.

Most dynamic reconstruction algorithms employ the information of an electrocardiogram (ECG) acquired synchronously with the X-ray images. With the ECG-signal, the heart phase of motion and rest can be identified. Only a subset of projections where the motion is neglectable are used to reconstruct one quasi-static state of the heart. However, the quality of these initial images is degraded due to the streak artifacts caused by angular undersampling and residual motion. Therefore, motion-compensated reconstruction algorithms are used, integrating the heart motion into the reconstruction and using all available projection images. Several motion estimation and compensation techniques or combined approaches exist and a short overview is given in Chapter 2. The last part covers the difference of cardiac chamber to cardiac vasculature reconstruction algorithms and presents the challenges of three-dimensional heart chamber reconstruction in clinical practice.

Chapter 3 Surface-based Motion Estimation, Reconstruction and Analysis

In this chapter, the focus is on the tomographic reconstruction and motion analysis of the left ventricle with a short acquisition. As previously described, the quality of the initial ECG-gated reconstructed volumes is hampered by streak artifacts due to the angular undersampling or even impossible since the number of projection images is limited. A motion estimation technique is presented based on dynamic left ventricular surface meshes extracted from the 2-D segmented bloodpool. As initialization, a surface mesh is fitted to the standard FDK reconstructed volume using all projection images. Then, the 2-D segmented bloodpool is used to detect the heart phase of each projection image. The projection images belonging to a certain heart phase are used to deform the initial surface mesh to the current heart phase. In order to perform a motion-compensated reconstruction, a dense motion vector field is required. Therefore, different interpolation techniques are used to map the sparse motion field defined on the surface control points to a dense motion vector field. Furthermore, it is possible to analyze the motion of the left ventricle using the left ventricular surface meshes. Functional parameters used for the analysis from other modalities are adapted to the C-arm CT mesh. Thus, the method has the potential to provide 3-D functional information directly in the interventional catheter lab which is not possible today. The last sections cover the evaluation of the methods, as well as the clinical challenges and a short summary.

Chapter 4 Volume-based Motion Estimation and Reconstruction

In contrary to the previous chapter, the focus is on the tomographic reconstruction of the whole heart based on a single sweep scan protocol without surface models to visualize the cardiac chambers. In comparison to the previous chapter, a longer scan and a different contrast protocol are used to visualize the whole heart. With the new imaging protocol, the quality of the retrospective ECG-gated reconstructions is increased and these volumes provide the possibility to use them as basis for cardiac motion estimation. Three different volume-based cardiac motion estimation approaches are presented utilizing multi-dimensional image registration techniques. One technique incorporated cyclic constraints into the registration process, the second approach combines the initial volume for registration and the last registration approach uses a deformable B-spline registration with different pre-processing steps. The methods are analyzed with respect to their computational complexity for comparison. In the evaluation section, the algorithms were quantitatively tested on simulated phantom datasets, as well as on clinical porcine models. The end of the chapter covers first patient results and a summary and conclusions section.

Chapter 5 Summary and Outlook

The last chapter provides a summary of the investigated approaches, conducted research and the scientific progress achieved by the work performed in this thesis. The chapter concludes with challenges and limitations of the presented contributions which open up new research topics and directions for further investigations.

.

CHAPTER 2

State-of-the-Art in 3-D Cardiac Imaging

2.1 General Notation of Reconstruction Algorithms 16

2.2 Static Image Reconstruction 16

2.3 From Static to Dynamic Image Reconstruction. 23

2.4 Motion Estimation Techniques 26

2.5 Motion-Compensated Image Reconstruction. 28

2.6 Joint Motion Estimation and Compensation. 30

2.7 Difference to Cardiac Vasculature Image Reconstruction 30

2.8 Challenges in Clinical Applications 32

2.9 Summary and Conclusions 32

Nowadays, 2-D angiography is the standard of reference for imaging and guidance of cardiac interventions using a C-arm system. Additionally, these systems provide the possibility of 3-D imaging. C-arm CT reconstructions of dynamic objects are quite challenging, however in some clinical procedures, e.g., pulmonary vein isolation and pulmonary artery interventions, standard 3-D reconstructions without motion compensation have proven to be useful, despite a slight motion blur, since these are relatively static structures [Nlke 10, Schw 11].

In recent years, various approaches have been presented in the field of motion-compensated cardiac vasculature reconstruction using C-arm CT [Blon 06, Hans 09, Rohk 10b, Schw 13]. Up to now, the reconstruction of cardiac chambers using an angiographic system is not widespread among the research groups [Laur 06, Prmm 09b, Thri 12c, Mory 14]. Therefore, in this chapter an overview of dynamic cardiac imaging beyond C-arm CT is provided. Throughout this chapter and thesis, the mathematical description is based on the notation introduced by Rohkohl [Rohk 10a]. In the first section, Section 2.1, the basic notation and geometry of the C-arm system is formally introduced, followed by a summary of state-of-the-art techniques for reconstruction of static 3-D objects with a C-arm CT in Section 2.2. In Section 2.3, techniques to map the reconstruction problem of dynamic objects to the reconstruction formulation of static objects are presented. The most popular approach utilizes an electrocardiogram (ECG)-signal acquired synchronous with the acquisition in order to use only the projection data belonging to a certain motion state. This results in a sparse angular sampling of the available projection data. Therefore, several techniques are deployed to estimate the motion by different motion estimation strategies in Section 2.4, and perform motion-compensated reconstructions, presented in Section 2.5 to make use of all acquired projection data. Instead of performing the motion estimation and compensation step sequentially, both steps can also be performed concurrently, see Section 2.6. Section 2.7 explains the differences between cardiac vasculature and cardiac chamber reconstruction. The chapter ends by pointing out the clinical challenges of cardiac imaging with an interventional C-arm system in Section 2.8 and the summary of this chapter is provided in Section 2.9.

2.1   General Notation of Reconstruction Algorithms

In this section the basic definition of the term reconstruction is explained, which is needed throughout this thesis.

The reconstruction formulas can be written as a function

$$f \; : \; \mathbb{R}^3 \times \mathbb{R}^{K_s} \mapsto \mathbb{R}, \tag{2.1}$$

where $f(\boldsymbol{x}, \boldsymbol{s})$ returns the reconstructed object value for a spatial three-dimensional location (voxel) with $\boldsymbol{x} \in \mathbb{R}^3$, $\boldsymbol{x} = (x_1, x_2, x_3)^T$ and a K_s-dimensional vector of real-valued parameters $\boldsymbol{s} \in \mathbb{R}^{K_s}$. The vector $\boldsymbol{s}$ includes parameters to represent the object as well as the motion model and varies from algorithm to algorithm and will be explained accordingly in the sections used.

The basic C-arm CT geometry is illustrated in Figure 2.1. Parameter S denotes the X-ray source. The detector origin is denoted with O, and $\boldsymbol{u} \in \mathbb{R}^2$, $\boldsymbol{u} = (u_1, u_2)^T$ is the position vector on the detector plane. The orthogonal projection of S is given by $\boldsymbol{u}_S$ on the detector. The origin of the 3-D world-coordinate system is set in reference to the C-arm isocenter I, i.e. the center of rotation. The rotation axis is oriented along x_3.

2.2   Static Image Reconstruction

A short review of the necessary details regarding cone-beam reconstruction for static objects is provided. Most of the motion-compensated reconstructions are adaptations of the static reconstruction algorithms.

Medical image reconstruction algorithms are of a complex nature and several modified algorithms for specific tasks and applications are published every year. In this thesis, we confine the introduction of reconstruction algorithms to the relevant parts needed. An extensive overview of the theory of reconstruction algorithms and their details can be found in the literature [Kak 99, Dsse 99, Buzu 08, Zeng 09, Shaw 14].

The family of reconstruction algorithms can be divided into three major groups: analytical, iterative reconstruction and geometric methods. Geometric reconstructions are a special type of reconstructions. In this case, the algorithms provide structural and morphological information instead of tomographic reconstructions. The different algorithms are now explained in more detail.

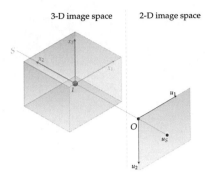

Figure 2.1: Geometry of a C-arm CT system and the corresponding coordinate systems. Parameter S denotes the X-ray source, the detector origin is denoted with O, and the orthogonal projection of S is given by u_S on the detector. The origin of the 3-D world-coordinate system is I.

2.2.1   Analytical Cone-beam Image Reconstruction

For analytical reconstruction, a function is given explicitly, describing the relationship between the reconstructed object attenuation value and the acquired projections. Due to the geometry of the system, different mappings or functions are required. Most of the reconstruction algorithms differ in their accuracy and practical applicability [Tuy 83, Gran 91, Kats 03, Noo 07]. In today's available C-arm CT scanners, an approximate cone-beam algorithm named after the inventors Feldkamp, Davis and Kress (FDK) is applied [Feld 84]. It is an extension of the widely used filtered-backprojection (FBP) fan-beam algorithm to 3-D cone-beam geometry. It produces acceptable results in clinical practice with a low computational effort compared to exact or iterative reconstruction algorithms. The reconstruction of a volume with the FDK formula is given in a discrete version with respect to the projection number i by

$$h_{\mathrm{FDK}}(i, \boldsymbol{x}) = w_D(i, \boldsymbol{x}) \cdot p_F(i, B(i, \boldsymbol{x})), \tag{2.2}$$

$$p_F(i, \boldsymbol{u}) = C \cdot \sum_k \Big(p(i, (k, u_2)^T) \cdot c(i, \boldsymbol{u}) \Big) \star g(u_1 - k), \tag{2.3}$$

$$f(\boldsymbol{x}, \cdot) = \sum_{i=1}^{N} h_{\mathrm{FDK}}(i, \boldsymbol{x}). \tag{2.4}$$

The index i denotes the i-th projection image, the function $w_D : \mathbb{N} \times \mathbb{R}^3 \mapsto \mathbb{R}$ is the distance weight of the FDK formula and based on the distance from source-to-detector and source-to-object. The pre-processed, filtered and redundancy weighted projection data is denoted as function $p_F : \mathbb{N} \times \mathbb{R}^2 \to \mathbb{R}$, where $p_F(i, \boldsymbol{u})$ returns the value of the i-th projection image at the position $\boldsymbol{u}$. The position $\boldsymbol{u}$ is determined by the perspective projection $B : \mathbb{N} \times \mathbb{R}^3 \mapsto \mathbb{R}^2$ with $B(i, \boldsymbol{x}) = \boldsymbol{u}$. The function $h_{\mathrm{FDK}}(i, \boldsymbol{x})$ denotes the i-th distance-weighted and pre-processed projection value contributing to value x. The function $c : \mathbb{N} \times \mathbb{R}^2 \mapsto \mathbb{R}$ describes the cosine and redundancy weighting of the pre-processed projection data, given by the function $p : \mathbb{N} \times \mathbb{R}^2 \mapsto \mathbb{R}$, where $p(i, u)$ returns the pre-processed value of the i-th projection image at the position u. The number of projection images is given by N. The redundancy weighting is required as a C-arm covers an angular range of about $\pi + 2 \cdot$ (fan angle) for a circular short-scan trajectory [Park 82]. C is a scaling constant and dependent on the scanner geometry [Rohk 08]. The function $g(n)$ describes the filtering kernel, an example is the row-wise 1-D Ram-Lak filter [Zeng 09]

$$g(n) = \begin{cases} \frac{1}{4}, & n = 0 \\ 0, & n \text{ even} \\ \frac{-1}{n^2 \pi^2}, & n \text{ odd.} \end{cases} \tag{2.5}$$

In this thesis, no physical effects are considered and hence the term pre-processed projection data means that line integrals are given at this point. As mentioned before, the position u is determined by the perspective projection $B : \mathbb{N} \times \mathbb{R}^3 \mapsto \mathbb{R}^2$ with $B(i, x) = u$. If the mapping to the detector coordinate u is at a non-integer pixel position, the value is computed by bilinear interpolation. The perspective mapping needs to be calibrated for each projection angle for a specific trajectory [Roug 93, Nava 98, Wies 00].

2.2.2 Iterative Image Reconstruction

Instead of describing the relation between a 3-D reconstruction and the projection data in an analytic form, a 3-D reconstruction can be alternatively achieved by optimization of an objective function. Assuming that a perfect 3-D reconstruction for a set of 2-D projection images is given, the forward projections (also called digitally reconstructed radiographs (DRRs)) should match the originally acquired projection data [Buzu 08]. Therefore, an optimization problem can be defined in order to minimize the difference between the DRRs of the reconstructed volume and the original projection data. The reconstruction problem can be defined as a system of linear equations. In practice, however, more projection data are available than voxels to be reconstructed. Hence, the system of linear equations is overdetermined and cannot be solved by direct methods, such as matrix inversion [Dsse 99]. Consequently, the optimal solution is found iteratively by optimization of an objective function, e.g., by using a gradient descent optimizer [Rohk 10a].

For iterative image reconstruction, the object needs to be represented by a set of basis functions. There exist different types of basis functions in order to represent the 3-D image, e.g., discrete grid voxels [Buzu 08], spherically symmetric basis functions (blobs) [Lewi 92, Mate 96] or new designed basis functions [Noo 12, Schm 12]. In this thesis notation, the representation of the basis functions is stored in the parameter vector $s \in \mathbb{R}^K$, in which all necessary basis function parameters are stored together, and named s_{im}. Here, the object is represented by voxel-based basis functions. The value at a voxel is then computed by the image representation $f(x, s)$ at the position $x \in \mathbb{R}^3$ with the parameters s. The DRR value of the reconstructed value $f(x, s)$ is

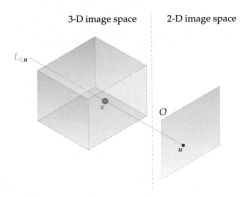

Figure 2.2: Illustration of the relation between the 3-D image space and the 2-D projection space. The pixel position u is the projection of x along the line $L_{i,u}$ for the i-th projection according to $B(i, x)$. O denotes the detector origin.

given by $r(i, u, s)$ with $r : \mathbb{N} \times \mathbb{R}^2 \times \mathbb{R}^K \mapsto \mathbb{R}$, with the position $u \in \mathbb{R}^2$ in the i-th projection image. In order to generate the DRR value,

$$r(i, u, s) = \sum_{x} A(i, x) \cdot f(x, s), \qquad (2.6)$$

with the function $A : \mathbb{N} \times \mathbb{R}^3 \mapsto \mathbb{R}$ returning a view angle and ray dependent weight according to the contribution of the position x to the observed line integral. Or in the case of a discrete reconstruction, the contribution to the sum of the line is returned. In the literature, these weights are often called system matrix, where the entries describe the contribution of each position to the line integral measured at the detector [Buzu 08]. There exist various approaches to define these contributions, e.g., as a simple binary mask if the ray crosses a voxel or not [Gord 70], as a ratio between intersection area and the voxel volume [Shep 82] or with the length of the intersection with the voxel [Sidd 85]. In this thesis, a ray casting approach is used similar to [Wein 08, Sche 11]. Hence, the DRR value is given as

$$r(i, u, s) = \sum_{x \in L_{i,u}} f(x, s), \qquad (2.7)$$

where $L_{i,u} = \{x \in \mathbb{R}^3 \,|\, B(i, x) = u\}$ defines the ray from the detector pixel u and projection image i to the X-ray source S. Only the measurement values along this ray are considered. For the voxel-based object representation, the value $f(x, s)$ along the ray $L_{i,u}$ is computed by trilinear interpolation [Jose 82]. An illustration of the relation between 3-D image space and 2-D projection space is given in Figure 2.2.

2.2.2.1   Non-constrained Iterative Image Reconstruction

In order to formulate the optimization strategy of an unconstrained iterative recon-
struction algorithm, an objective function $\mathcal{L} : \mathbb{R}^K \mapsto \mathbb{R}$ needs to be defined, i.e.

$$\hat{s}_{\text{im}} = \underset{s_{\text{im}}}{\arg\min}\, \mathcal{L}(s_{\text{im}}), \qquad \text{where} \qquad (2.8)$$

$$\mathcal{L}(s_{\text{im}}) = \sum_{i=1}^{N} d(i, s). \qquad (2.9)$$

The function $d : \mathbb{N} \times \mathbb{R}^K \mapsto \mathbb{R}$ measures the dissimilarity of the i-th projection image
to the i-th DRR. The dissimilarity measure varies between different applications and
several can be found in the literature [Soti 13, Hahn 09, Mode 03].

2.2.2.2   Compressed Sensing as Constrained Iterative Image Reconstruction

In the literature, a particular type of constrained iterative reconstruction is also often
called compressed sensing (CS). The compressed sensing idea was first published
by Donoho [Dono 06] and Candès [Cand 06a, Cand 06b]. In general, compressive
sampling or compressed sensing deals with the recovery of signals or images from
fewer measurements than conventional methods. There is an extensive introduction
in the literature about the mathematical background from signal processing [Cand 07,
Cand 08, Zeng 09]. The basic idea for the adaptation to 3-D image reconstruction is,
a sparsified volume is reconstructed instead of the target volume, where the sparse
volume has significantly fewer non-zero voxels. Consequently, the sparsified volume
can be reconstructed from undersampled measurements without artifacts. After the
reconstruction of the sparse volume, the "inverse" of the sparsifying transform is
applied to obtain the target image. No explicit form of the "inverse" transform is
required in practice [Chen 08]. The basic formulation of a CS image reconstruction
problem is

$$\mathcal{L}(s_{\text{im}}) = ||\Psi f(x, s)||_1, \quad \text{s.t.} \sum_{i \in \mathcal{N}} d(i, s) < \epsilon^2, \qquad (2.10)$$

$$d(i, s) = \sum_{u} (p(i, u) - r(i, u, s))^2. \qquad (2.11)$$

The sparsifying transform is denoted as Ψ and $||f(x, s)||_1 = \sum_x |f(x, s)|$ is the
l_1−norm of the function values of $f(x, s)$. The objective function $\mathcal{L}(s_{\text{im}})$ is minimized subject to the data constraint, where the DRRs of the reconstruction need
to fit to a subset $\mathcal{N} \subset N$ of the original measured projection images. The upper
bound of the data error is given by ϵ^2. Various sparsifying transforms are known in
the literature, e.g., discrete gradient transforms [Sidk 06, Sidk 08], or wavelet transforms [Lust 07]. For cardiac chamber and coronary artery imaging, there exist also
approaches which additionally take into account temporal similarity between successive heart phases [Lang 12, Mory 14]. In general, various optimization schemes exist
and the optimization schemes can vary.

Prior Image Constrained Compressed Sensing (PICCS). In compressed
sensing applications, the number of projections $i \in \mathcal{N}$, with $\mathcal{N} \subset N$ in Equation

(2.11), which enforce the data consistency, are limited. The resulting volumes have a low signal-to-noise (SNR) ratio. In order to improve the resulting SNR of the reconstruction, a prior image is introduced in the optimization to inherit the high SNR value of the prior volume [Chen 08]. This approach was published as prior image constrained compressed sensing algorithm (PICCS) by Chen et al. [Chen 08]. The PICCS objective function was originally stated as a constrained minimization problem

$$\hat{s}_{\text{im}} = \underset{s_{\text{im}}}{\arg\min} \, \mathcal{L}(s_{\text{im}}), \quad \text{s.t.} \sum_{i \in \mathcal{N}} d(i, s) < \epsilon^2 \quad \text{with} \tag{2.12}$$

$$\mathcal{L}(s_{\text{im}}) = \alpha \cdot ||\Psi_1 \left(f(x, s) - f_P(x) \right)||_1 + (1 - \alpha) \cdot ||\Psi_2 f(x, s)||_1, \tag{2.13}$$

where $\alpha \in [0, 1]$ is the control parameter. When $\alpha = 0$, the PICCS algorithm reduces to the conventional CS algorithm stated in Equation (2.10). The prior image is denoted as $f_P(x)$ and is usually reconstructed by a standard FDK algorithm as described in Section 2.2.1 using all acquired projection data. The sparsifying transforms Ψ_1 and Ψ_2 can be chosen arbitrarily. One common example of a sparsifying transform is the discrete gradient transform given by

$$||\Psi f(x, s)||_1 = \sum_x \sqrt{\varepsilon + \sum_j \left(\frac{\partial f(x, s)}{\partial s_j} \right)^2}. \tag{2.14}$$

This function is also known as total variation (TV). The parameter ε is needed for a robust analytical derivative of the objective function to avoid singularities at the origin. This approach is controversially discussed in the literature [Boyd 04]. The PICCS objective function is then given as

$$\mathcal{L}(s_{\text{im}}) = \alpha \cdot \sum_x \sqrt{\varepsilon + \sum_j \left(\frac{\partial \left(f - f_P \right) (x, s)}{\partial s_j} \right)^2}$$

$$+ (1 - \alpha) \cdot \sum_x \sqrt{\varepsilon + \sum_j \left(\frac{\partial f(x, s)}{\partial s_j} \right)^2}. \tag{2.15}$$

In most publications, the optimization problem is solved iteratively using an alternating minimization procedure. First, the data consistency term is optimized to reconstruct an initial image, as described in Section 2.2.2 to fulfill Equation (2.10). Then, the objective function is minimized by a gradient descent method [Chen 08, Nett 08a, Chen 12]. The optimization problem can also be formulated as a non-constrained optimization problem [Rami 11, Thri 12a, Thri 12b, Thri 12c, Thri 13].

Improved Total Variation. As presented in the previous paragraph, the optimization strategy for the constrained problem is often performed separately in an alternating manner. Therefore, in order to increase convergence speed, it needs to be ensured that the data consistency term reduces to an optimal value while the

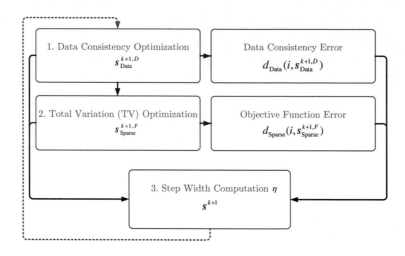

Figure 2.3: Schematic overview of the improved total variation (iTV) algorithm.

objective function value is kept at a low level [Rits 10]. The parameter ϵ in Equations (2.10) and (2.12), characterizes the data consistency and the optimal value ϵ_{opt} needs to be known beforehand. It depends on physical effects, like scatter, beam hardening, and misalignment in the data and noise. If ϵ is not chosen to be close to ϵ_{opt} the influence of the objective function increases. If ϵ is chosen too small, the impact of the objective function decreases. A discussion on this can be found in [Bian 10]. The key problem is that the objective function and the data consistency term are defined in different domains. Therefore, the step-size determination of both optimization procedures needs to be transferred to the projection data domain and adapted to each other. This algorithm is called improved total variation (iTV) introduced by Ritschl et al. [Rits 11]. The object parameters $s_{\text{Data}} \in \mathbb{R}^{K_{\text{Data}}}$, and $f_{\text{Data}}(x, s_{\text{Data}})$ returning the value of the iterative reconstructed object at voxel position x and a parameter set $s_{\text{Sparse}} \in \mathbb{R}^{K_{\text{Sparse}}}$, with $f_{\text{Sparse}}(x, s_{\text{Sparse}})$ returning the object value of the optimized object at the 3-D position x are defined. The overall optimized parameters $s^{k+1} \in \mathbb{R}^{K_S}$ with $k = \{1, \ldots, O\}$ outer iterations (minimization of the data consistency term and the objective function) are given as

$$s^{k+1} = (1 - \eta) \cdot s_{\text{Data}}^{k+1,D} + \eta \cdot s_{\text{Sparse}}^{k+1,F}, \qquad (2.16)$$

where D denotes the data consistency and F the sparse-optimized iterations. The parameter $\eta \in]0, 1]$ is used to adapt the TV step size in the 3-D image domain. However, the data error is defined in 2-D projection space, therefore, another parameter $\omega_{\text{iTV}} \in]0, 1]$ is introduced in 2-D projection space, weighting the 2-D data error accordingly, to find parameters s_{Data} and s_{Sparse} leading to the defined 2-D errors. Due to the linearity of the X-ray transform, and the knowledge that the TV of the function $f(\boldsymbol{x}, \boldsymbol{s}^{k+1})$ is reduced for all η [Rits 11], the step size η can be determined by solving the following quadratic equation

$$\sum_{i \in \mathcal{N}} d(i, \boldsymbol{s}^{k+1}) = (1 - \omega_{\text{iTV}}) \sum_{i \in \mathcal{N}} d_{\text{Data}}(i, \boldsymbol{s}_{\text{Data}}^{k+1,D}) + \omega_{\text{iTV}} \sum_{i \in \mathcal{N}} d(i, \boldsymbol{s}^{k}), \qquad (2.17)$$

where $\sum_{i \in \mathcal{N}} d(i, \boldsymbol{s}^{k+1})$ denotes the error between the DRRs and the original measured projections at the outer iteration $k + 1$ from the volume $f(\boldsymbol{x}, \boldsymbol{s}^{k+1})$, $\sum_{i \in \mathcal{N}} d_{\text{Data}}(i, \boldsymbol{s}_{\text{Data}}^{k+1,D})$ is the data error after D data consistency iterations and $\sum_{i \in \mathcal{N}} d(i, \boldsymbol{s}^{k})$ is the error at the previous iteration k , i.e. after D data consistency and F TV optimization steps. The parameter η needs to be reset to 1 if $\eta > 1$ is a possible solution [Rits 11]. The parameter ω_{iTV} needs to be set by the user. A schematic overview of the whole iTV algorithm can be found in Figure 2.3.

2.2.3   Geometric Image Reconstruction

The last group of reconstruction algorithms is the field of geometric reconstructions. In the literature, several approaches to recover the 3-D shape of the left ventricle with biplane X-ray systems are described. When using a biplane system, the epipolar constraint [Hart 04] can be exploited in order to compute the 3-D left ventricle (LV) shape from two orthogonal simultaneously acquired projection images. Backfrieder et al. [Back 05] proposed to deform initial super ellipses until their projection profiles optimally fit to the measured projections. The generated model can be used to perform an LV wall motion analysis [Swob 05]. A similar approach is used in Medina et al. and Mantilla et al. [Medi 06, Mant 08], where ellipsoidal approximations derived from the input ventriculograms are deformed to match the input projections. Other approaches make use of multi-view cardiograms to improve the accuracy of the LV shapes. Moriyama et al. [Mori 02] proposed an iterative framework to recover LV meshes from multi views by fitting a dynamic surface model defined by B-splines to the LV. All of the previously mentioned approaches make use of the synchronously acquired orthogonal ventriculograms from a biplane system. For a rotating C arm CT system, no projections of the same heart phase in the same heart cycle are acquired synchronously, and hence, no 3-D point correspondences can be established by the epipolar constraint. Most of the presented work utilizes ellipsoidal structures for the reconstruction of the LV. This assumption may not hold for pathological LVs, e.g., after a myocardial infarct [Gutb 13]. Therefore, more degrees of freedom for the surface generation can improve the reconstruction of the dynamic LV surface. A review on geometric modeling and reconstruction for different imaging modalities can be found in Frangi et al. [Fran 01].

2.3   From Static to Dynamic Image Reconstruction using ECG-Gating

In order to increase the temporal resolution and minimize the imaging artifacts in cardiac imaging due to the motion, only a subset of the projections belonging to

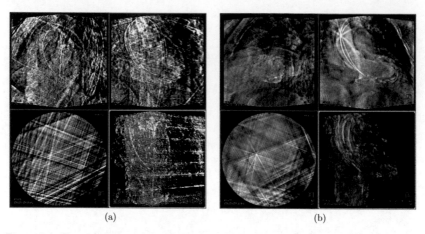

(a)   (b)

Figure 2.4: Example image of an ECG-gated reconstruction of a left ventricle from a 5 s scan, a heart rate of 58.3±0.3 bpm, with the following parameters: (a) $\phi_r = 0.75$, $w \to 0$ and $\vartheta = 0$ resulting in a total of 5 projections. Only streaks are visible in the reconstruction and no structure is reconstructed. (b) $\phi_r = 0.75$, $w = 0.4$ and $\vartheta = 4$ resulting in a total of 54 weighted projections. The left ventricle is superposed by streak artifacts and no clear endocardial structure can be delineated. The image data was provided by Dr. med. Schultz from the Thoraxcenter, Erasmus MC Rotterdam, The Netherlands.

that specific motion state are used for reconstruction. Therefore, the dynamic reconstruction problem is reduced to a static reconstruction problem. There exist either prospective [Guru 08] or retrospective [Desj 04] electrocardiogram (ECG)-gating approaches. The latter approach is less sensitive to heart rate changes than the prospective approach, however, at the expense of a higher radiation dose. The basic principle of retrospective ECG-gating and two different reconstruction techniques are described below.

An electrocardiogram (ECG)-signal is acquired synchronously with the image acquisition. The single heart phase for each time step is then computed by linear interpolation between two successive R-peaks in the ECG signal. In order to reconstruct a certain heart phase, only those projections are considered for which the heart phase is close to the cardiac phase of interest [Desj 04]. The closeness of two heart phases ϕ_1 and ϕ_2 is given according to Rohkohl [Rohk 10a] by the distance function $d_\phi : [0, 1] \times [0, 1] \to [0, 1]$

$$d_\phi(\phi_1, \phi_2) = \min_{\zeta \in \{0, 1, -1\}} |\phi_1 - \phi_2 + \zeta|. \qquad (2.18)$$

2.3.1 Single Sweep ECG-Gated Image Reconstruction

A single sweep acquisition means that only one rotation of the C-arm around the patient is performed. For a single sweep ECG-gated reconstruction, a weighting function $\lambda : \mathbb{N} \times \mathbb{R}^3 \mapsto [0, 1]$ is introduced, that assigns an impact weight to each image on the reconstruction result. The heart phase is denoted with $\phi \in [0,1]$ and the relative heart phase of the i-th projection image is given by $\phi(i)$. The gating function λ is parametrized by a vector $\boldsymbol{s}_{\mathrm{ga}} = (\phi_r, w, \vartheta)^\top$ with the reference heart phase $\phi_r \in [0,1]$, the phase-width $w \in (0,1]$ and the shape-parameter $\vartheta \in [0,\infty)$. The gating function $\lambda(i, \boldsymbol{s}_{\mathrm{ga}})$ returns the gating weight. The weighting function is centered at a specific heart phase ϕ_r and can have the shape of a cosine [Rohk 08] or a rectangular window [Schf 06]. A general definition of the weighting function is given accordingly to [Rohk 10a] by

$$\lambda(i, \boldsymbol{s}_{\mathrm{ga}}) = \begin{cases} \cos^\vartheta \left(\frac{d_\phi(\phi(i),\phi_r)}{w} \pi \right) & , \text{ if } d_\phi(\phi(i),\phi_r) \le \frac{w}{2} \\ 0 & \text{ otherwise.} \end{cases} \qquad (2.19)$$

The function $f_{\phi_k}(\boldsymbol{x}, \boldsymbol{s})$ returns the reconstructed object at the 3-D position $\boldsymbol{x}$ and the heart phase $\phi_k \in \{1, \ldots, K\}$, where K denotes a certain number of heart phases to be reconstructed. The heart phase ϕ_k corresponds to a relative heart phase of $\phi \in [0,1]$. Hence, different heart phases can be reconstructed with data from one C-arm rotation by

$$f_{\phi_k}(\boldsymbol{x}, \boldsymbol{s}) = \sum_{i=1}^{N} \lambda(i, \boldsymbol{s}_{\mathrm{ga}}) \cdot h_{\mathrm{FDK}}(i, \boldsymbol{x}) \qquad (2.20)$$

$$= \sum_{i=1}^{N} h_{\mathrm{gFDK}}(i, \boldsymbol{x}, \boldsymbol{s}_{\mathrm{ga}}). \qquad (2.21)$$

Since a small number of cardiac cycles are observed during a single rotation of a C-arm system, which lasts between 5 s and 15 s, only a small number of projection images are available for the reconstruction of one heart phase. For example, if the rotation duration is 5 s and the patient has a heart rate of 60 bpm, and $w \to 0$, i.e. nearest-neighbor gating and only 1 image per heart cycle, only 5 projections per heart phase are available. The ECG-gated images are of low quality and suffer from angular undersampling artifacts. In Figure 2.4, an example of an ECG-gated reconstruction of a left heart ventricle of a 5 s scan and a patient's heart rate of 58.3±0.3 bpm is given, with different parameter settings.

2.3.2   Multiple Sweep ECG-Gated Image Reconstruction

For the heart chambers, the ECG-gated projection data of a single sweep leads to prominent streak artifacts and a poor signal-to-noise ratio, cf. Figure 2.4. Consequently, multiple sweeps S_w in forward and backward direction of the C-arm can be performed to acquire enough projections for each heart phase. Projection data of several heart cycles can be combined to reconstruct images, which is also called multisegment reconstruction. Data acquired at different heart cycles should provide complementary coverage over the full angular range such that a complete dataset is obtained [Laur 06]. In order to reconstruct a single 3-D volume from the acquired dynamic data, projection images corresponding to the desired cardiac phase have to be extracted from the series of acquired forward and backward runs. Thus, for each angular position, only the projection acquired closest to the desired cardiac phase is used. Here, the heart phase is given by the function $\phi : \mathbb{N}^2 \to [0,1]$. The closeness of each current heart phase $\phi(i, s_w)$ to the reference heart phase ϕ_r is computed as described in Equation (2.18). Here, $i \in \{1, \ldots, N\}$ denotes the number of projections of one sweep and $s_w \in \{1, \ldots, S_w\}$ the total number of all forward and backward runs. Now, the weighting function $\lambda : \mathbb{N}^2 \times [0,1] \mapsto \{0,1\}$, returns the binary weight of the projection image i in the s_w-th run according to

$$\lambda(i, s_w, \phi_r) = \begin{cases} 1 & \text{, if } d_\phi(\phi(i, s_w), \phi_r) \leq \min_{s \in \{1, \ldots S_w\}} (d_\phi(\phi(i, s), \phi_r)) \\ 0 & \text{otherwise.} \end{cases} \quad (2.22)$$

The reconstruction is then defined by

$$f_{\phi_k}(\boldsymbol{x}, \boldsymbol{s}) = \sum_{s_w=1}^{S_w} \sum_{i=1}^{N} \lambda(i, s_w, \phi_r) \cdot h_{\text{FDK}}(i, s_w, \boldsymbol{x}) \quad (2.23)$$

$$= \sum_{s_w=1}^{S_w} \sum_{i=1}^{N} h_{\text{gFDK}}(i, s_w, \boldsymbol{x}, \phi_r), \quad (2.24)$$

where $h_{\text{FDK}}(i, s_w, \boldsymbol{x})$ denotes the i-th pre-processed projection value contributing to voxel $\boldsymbol{x}$ in the s_w-th sweep, cf. Section 2.2.1. With no temporal smoothing introduced, this will result in the highest temporal resolution possible with the available data. But, the longer imaging time of multiple runs results in a higher contrast burden and radiation dose for the patient. Furthermore, only a certain number of cardiac phases can be reconstructed depending on the number of sweeps [Laur 06, Prmm 09a].

2.4   Motion Estimation Techniques

A possible solution to improve the image quality is the use of all acquired projection data in combination with compensation for the cardiac motion in the reconstruction step. One possibility to estimate the motion is deformable image registration. Deformable registration is a fundamental task in medical image processing. Depending on the underlying image quality, defined by the used modalities for image acquisition and application, various optimization techniques and objective functions exist [Soti 13, Mkel 02]. Therefore, two challenging tasks need to be solved: (1) initial images need to be of good quality and (2) find a stable registration approach. A broad overview of deformable image registration was recently given by Sotiras et al. [Soti 13] and in particular for cardiac motion estimation in Mäkelä et al. [Mkel 02]. In the following subsections, different approaches for motion estimation are reviewed, which exhibit similarities to cardiac motion estimation with a C-arm CT.

2.4.1   3-D/3-D Image Registration

Cardiac motion estimation via 3-D/3-D image registration is already extensively investigated for other imaging modalities, like cardiac computed tomography (CT) [Tagu 08, Isol 10b], ultrasound (US) [Zhan 11] or cardiac magnetic resonance (MR) imaging [Perp 05]. The deformation between a reference heart phase and other heart phases is computed by various optimization routines. The individual algorithms differ in the used motion model, objective function, constraints, and optimization techniques. In Isola et al. [Isol 10a], a fully automatic registration for recovery of a motion vector field for cardiac CT with a multi-resolution and adapted optimization routine was proposed. The cardiac motion is represented by cubic B-splines [Unse 99, Rcke 99] and the sum of squared differences (SSD) was used as similarity measure. The optimization is done with a stochastic gradient descent of Robbins-Monro [Robb 51]. A similar approach was presented by Tang et al. [Tang 12, Tang 13], the cardiac motion is modeled by cubic B-splines, the weighted least-squared difference is used as objective function and optimized by an iterative nested conjugate gradient.

In the field of motion estimation for cone beam CT, some approaches deal with respiratory motion during radiotherapy procedures. In Brehm et al. [Breh 12] different respiratory-gated images are registered to each other by a demon's algorithm and cyclic constraints are introduced to lower the influence of the undersampling streak artifacts. An extension of this approach utilizes a patient specific artifact model to improve the registration result [Breh 13]. Another approach computes an intermediate volume with low spatial but high temporal resolution. From this dataset, principal components are extracted, which represent the temporal variation [Chri 13]. These principal components are used to reconstruct an intermediate volume with full spatial and temporal resolution. On this data, optical flow registration is applied to estimate the motion and finally to compensate for it.

All proposed approaches have initial images of sufficient quality or employ strategies to improve the image quality before the registration. The motion estimation result is highly dependent on the quality of the initial reconstructed images [Mlle 12a]. Especially in cardiac C-arm CT, the initial images, e.g., based on retrospective single sweep ECG-gating, suffer from temporal undersampling and the image quality is highly degraded by streak artifacts. Furthermore, the reconstruction of several images with equivalent good quality is problematic. Mostly the mid-systolic phase is more challenging to reconstruct due to the fast movement of the coronaries and the cardiac chambers [Prmm 06b, Husm 07, Rohk 08]. Up to now, there exists one 3-D/3-D registration approach for cardiac C-arm CT data. In Prümmer et al. [Prmm 09b, Prmm 09a], a multiple sweep cardiac protocol is used and different heart phases are reconstructed as described in Section 2.3.2. The motion is estimated by minimizing the SSD between the volumes applying various regularizations.

2.4.2   2-D/3-D Image Registration

As described in Section 2.4.1, for the 3-D/3-D image registration approach, initial reconstructed volumes of equivalent good image quality are required in order to estimate the motion. A 2-D/3-D image registration approach has the advantage that only one volume of satisfactory image quality is needed. The goal of 2-D/3-D registration is to estimate the 3-D transformation of the reconstructed volume that aligns the 3-D volume with the measured 2-D images. The 2-D/3-D registration is often used to align pre-interventional images, e.g., CT or MR volumes with the interventional X-ray images for guidance of the physician [Prmm 06a, Wang 13b, Wang 13c]. Most of the approaches make use of an affine or rigid transformation. However, in some clinical applications it is more reasonable to describe the transformations by a free-form displacement field as in Prümmer et al. [Prmm 06a].

A challenging problem for 2-D/3-D registration for rotational angiography is presented by the overlapping structures in the 2-D projection images. Therefore, in order to estimate motion, e.g., from coronary arteries, most approaches use a geometric representation like their centerlines [Blon 06, Shec 03]. The motion model parameters in 3-D are adapted such that the transformed centerlines for one heart phase, match the centerlines in the 2-D projection images.

2.4.3   2-D/2-D Image Registration

In general, a 2-D/2-D motion estimation algorithm cannot be applied directly to the 2-D projection images, since the heart and its coronaries are moving rapidly during a C-arm CT scan and overlapping structures can mislead the registration. Up to now, it has only been applied to the motion estimation of sparse high contrast structures such as coronary arteries. Hansis et al. [Hans 08b] proposed alignment of the 2-D vessel centerlines from an initial ECG-gated reconstruction to the 2-D centerlines detected in the original projection images. The 2-D and 3-D centerline detection, however, is a challenging task and the registration result is highly dependent on the segmentation.

For small residual motion, Schwemmer et al. [Schw 13] proposed a 2-D/2-D registration method for coronary motion estimation and compensation. The mapping of the forward projections of an initial ECG-gated reconstruction to the original projections belonging to the same heart phase is performed by a deformable B-spline registration with normalized cross correlation as objective function. A successive motion-compensated reconstruction results in a sharper 3-D reconstruction with improved image quality without the need to extract centerlines.

Both presented methods require pre-processing steps in order to eliminate structures not belonging to the vasculature in the 2-D projection images. For the cardiac chambers this is not applicable due to non homogenous contrast distribution inside the bloodpool and lower contrast inside the chambers compared to the sparse and high contrast coronaries.

2.5   Motion-Compensated Image Reconstruction

In general, there exist two kinds of motion-compensated reconstruction algorithms - one compensates for the estimated motion in the 2-D projection space and the second type compensates for the motion in the 3-D image space.

2.5.1   Motion Compensation in 2-D Projection Space

A motion-compensated reconstruction can be performed in the 2-D projection space by warping the original projection image to the digital forward projections of an initial reconstruction, e.g., of the coronary arteries. From the transformed projection data, an improved reconstruction can be computed [Hans 08b, Schw 13]. However, the amount of motion for which it is possible to compensate is limited.

2.5.2   Motion Compensation in 3-D Image Space

The 3-D motion compensation approach is more general and can be applied to various kinds of motion. The parameter vector $s \in \mathbb{R}^{K_S}$ contains real-valued parameters to represent the object. Now, the vector s is extended by parameters s_{mm} containing the parameters of the used motion model function. In general, the mapping from 3-D to 2-D space is deformed according to the motion model parameters. The adaptation of the reconstruction formulas for iterative and analytical reconstruction are derived in the following sections.

2.5.2.1   Iterative Algorithms

There exist a few techniques, which integrate the change of the projection operator directly into an iterative reconstruction framework. They deform the DRR generator according to the motion information [Blon 04, Blon 06, Hans 09]. Therefore, the dynamic DRR generator based on ray casting is reformulated to

$$r(i, \boldsymbol{u}, \boldsymbol{s}) = \sum_{\boldsymbol{x} \in L_{i,\boldsymbol{u}}} f(\underbrace{M(i, \boldsymbol{x}, \boldsymbol{s}_{\mathrm{mm}})}_{\boldsymbol{x}'}, \boldsymbol{s}), \qquad (2.25)$$

where the motion model function $M : \mathbb{N} \times \mathbb{R}^3 \times \mathbb{R}^{K_{\mathrm{mm}}} \mapsto \mathbb{R}^3$ maps the voxel position $\boldsymbol{x} \in \mathbb{R}^3$ to the new position $\boldsymbol{x}' \in \mathbb{R}^3$ according to given motion model parameters $\boldsymbol{s}_{\mathrm{mm}} \in \mathbb{R}^{K_{\mathrm{mm}}}$. The dynamic DRR generation needs to be propagated into the analytical derivative of the objective function for iterative image reconstruction Equation (2.8), which can be done accordingly to [Blon 06].

2.5.2.2   Analytic Algorithms

Integration of motion into the analytical reconstruction formula is not as straightforward as for the 2-D motion compensation case. It requires adaptation of the redundancy weights and the filtering step. One algorithm which integrated motion into the backprojection formula showed that it is possible to exactly compensate for transformations, larger than the affine class, in the backprojection step by adaptation of the filtering step [Desb 07]. However, the motion model allows only a mapping from lines onto lines and no free-form deformations. Taguchi et al. [Tagu 07, Tagu 08] presented motion-compensated reconstruction using locally varying affine transformations. For cardiac motion-compensated reconstruction, this kind of motion is not necessarily sufficient. An approximate reconstruction of the FDK formula was proposed in [Gran 02, Schf 06]. The estimated motion vector field is incorporated into a voxel-driven filtered backprojection reconstruction algorithm. The motion correction is applied during the backprojection step by shifting the voxel to be reconstructed according to the motion vector field. A schematic illustration of the motion-compensated backprojection is given in Figure 2.5. The motion model function $M : \mathbb{N} \times \mathbb{R}^3 \times \mathbb{R}^{K_{\mathrm{mm}}} \mapsto \mathbb{R}^3$ again maps the voxel position $\boldsymbol{x}$ to the new position $\boldsymbol{x}'$ according to given motion model parameters $\boldsymbol{s}_{\mathrm{mm}} \in \mathbb{R}^{K_{\mathrm{mm}}}$. The vectors $\boldsymbol{u}$ and $\boldsymbol{u}'$ are the perspective projections of $\boldsymbol{x}$ and $\boldsymbol{x}'$ given by $B(i, \boldsymbol{x}) = \boldsymbol{u}$ and $B(i, \boldsymbol{x}') = \boldsymbol{u}'$. Instead of accumulating the 2-D projection value at position $\boldsymbol{u}$ to the position $\boldsymbol{x}$, the value at $\boldsymbol{u}'$ is backprojected.

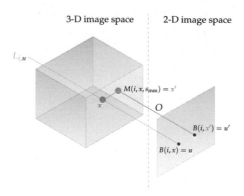

Figure 2.5: A simplified scheme of the voxel-based motion compensation. The detector origin is given by the the parameter O. Instead of the backprojection of u to the position x, the value u' corresponding to x' is used.

Formally, a motion-compensated FDK reconstruction is described by

$$f(\boldsymbol{x}, \boldsymbol{s}_{\mathrm{mm}}) \;=\; \sum_{i=1}^{N} w_D\big(i, \underbrace{M(i, \boldsymbol{x}, \boldsymbol{s}_{\mathrm{mm}})}_{\boldsymbol{x}'}\big) \cdot p_F\big(i, \underbrace{B\big(i, \underbrace{M(i, \boldsymbol{x}, \boldsymbol{s}_{\mathrm{mm}})}_{\boldsymbol{x}'}\big)}_{\boldsymbol{u}'}\big) \tag{2.26}$$

$$\;=\; \sum_{i=1}^{N} h_{\mathrm{FDK}}\big(i, M(i, \boldsymbol{x}, \boldsymbol{s}_{\mathrm{mm}})\big). \tag{2.27}$$

2.6   Joint Motion Estimation and Compensation

A challenging task is a combined approach for estimation and compensation of the motion. A few approaches introduce the motion estimation into the iterative reconstruction presented in Section 2.2.2. In addition to the unknown intensity values in the reconstructed volume, the motion model parameters need to be estimated [Scho 07, Chun 09, Hans 09, Camm 11, Wang 13a]. The number of unknowns increases the complexity of the optimization problem enormously. Consequently, the runtime of the optimization is prolonged and the optimization may get caught in a local minimum, i.e. a less optimal reconstruction quality is achieved [Rohk 10a].

2.7   Difference to Cardiac Vasculature Image Reconstruction Methods

Up to now, only a few publications are specifically approaching motion-compensated reconstruction of cardiac chambers with an interventional C-arm system [Laur 06,

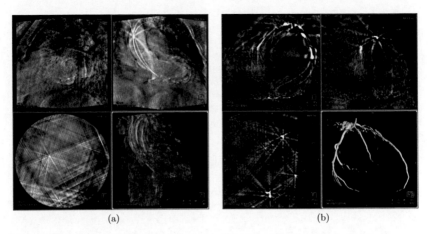

(a)   (b)

Figure 2.6: Example of ECG-gated reconstructions (a) of a left ventricle from a 5 s scan, a heart rate of 58.3±0.3 bpm, with the following parameters: $\phi_r = 0.75$, $w = 0.4$ and $\vartheta = 4$ resulting in a total of 54 weighted projections. The image data was provided by Dr. med. Schultz from the Thoraxcenter, Erasmus MC Rotterdam, The Netherlands. (b) of a left coronary artery from a 5 s scan, a heart rate of 64.3±1.9 bpm, with the following parameters: $\phi_r = 0.75$, $w = 0.4$ and $\vartheta = 4$ resulting in total of 52 weighted projections. The image data was provided by Prof. Dr. med. Böcker and Dr. med. Skurzewski, St. Marienhospital Hamm, Germany.

Prmm 09b, Prmm 09a, Thri 12c, Mory 14]. In contrast, considerable research has been published in the area of cardiac vasculature reconstruction [Hans 08a, Hans 09, Rohk 10b, Isol 12]. The main reasons for that are the high contrast and sparse structures, compared to the low contrast heart chambers with muscular texture. Therefore, some pre-processing steps which eliminate background structures around the coronaries in the 2-D X-ray images cannot be applied to cardiac chambers, e.g., morphological top hat filtering [Hans 08b, Hans 08a]. Also reduction of the undersampling artifacts in 3-D by a streak-reduced gated short-scan reconstruction [Rohk 08, Rohk 10b] cannot be used. Furthermore, the ECG-gated reconstructions of the coronaries in a quiet heart phase is of sufficient quality to use it, e.g., as initial image to estimate residual motion by 2-D/2-D registration approach [Schw 13]. Example ECG-gated reconstructions of a left heart ventricle and a left coronary artery using almost the same number of projection images are presented in Figure 2.6. It can be seen that the sparse and high contrast structure of coronaries can be recovered using the ECG-gated approach, compared to the heart chamber reconstruction. Some approaches also use the ECG-gated reconstruction to detect geometric features like the center-lines of the coronaries for motion estimation [Hans 08b, Hans 08a]. Consequently, motion estimation and compensation algorithms presented in the literature for cardiac vasculature reconstruction cannot be used for reconstruction of non-sparse and low contrast objects such as cardiac chambers.

2.8 Challenges in Clinical Applications

One main challenge in cardiac chamber reconstruction with an interventional C-arm system is the long acquisition time. The scanning time lies between 5 s and 15 s. Only a few hundred projection images are acquired, which is significantly lower than for conventional CT systems. Consequently, retrospective ECG-gating results in highly undersampled reconstructed volumes with severe streak artifacts, cf. Figures 2.4 and 2.6. The percentage of undersampling is defined by the patient's heart rate, the imaging frame rate and the scanning duration. The scan time cannot be arbitrarily prolonged since the patient is exposed to X-rays and iodinated contrast agent has to be administered continuously in order to visualize the bloodpool of the heart. The total amount of injected contrast agent needs to be reduced, therefore, the contrast that is achieved is not nearly as high as that seen in the coronary arteries. The image acquisition and contrast protocol needs to be evaluated for 3-D imaging of the heart chambers with the C-arm CT system using one single scan. The applied reconstruction algorithms are highly dependent on the clinical acquisition.

2.9 Summary and Conclusions

In this chapter, a short summary of the state-of-the-art reconstruction algorithms for cone-beam reconstruction was given. Since dynamic imaging of cardiac chambers with a C-arm CT is a quite new and challenging task, up to now, only a limited number of publications and research teams tackle this problem. Therefore, the review of dynamic reconstruction techniques is beyond cardiac C-arm CT and covers relevant publications, which deal with similar problems. Due to the long acquisition time, the motion of the cardiac chambers must be taken into account in the 3-D tomographic reconstruction step. The number of the acquired high resolution projection images is limited to a few hundred. Consequently, retrospective ECG-gated reconstructed volumes suffer from streak artifacts, noise, and residual motion. The amount of undersampling is dependent on the specific acquisition protocol, the imaging framerate, and the heart rate of the patient. The generation of initial and useful 3-D images for motion estimation by deformable registration is quite challenging. Consequently, motion estimation techniques from other modalities, e.g., CT cannot be directly applied to the data from C-arm CT. Additionally, algorithms developed for cardiac vasculature reconstruction make different assumptions which do not hold for cardiac chamber reconstruction. The chambers do not have sparse and high contrast structure such as the coronaries, hence, some pre-processing steps assuming high contrast objects are not feasible here. Prior work for motion-compensated reconstruction of cardiac chambers using a C-arm CT was done by Lauritsch et al. [Laur 06] and Prümmer et al. [Prmm 09b]. They used a multi-sweep protocol of the C-arm and selected for each viewing angle the projection closest to the reference heart phase. In this thesis, cardiac protocols based on one C-arm rotation are used and consequently, new reconstruction techniques are required for cardiac chambers using C-arm CT data.

CHAPTER 3

Surface-based Motion Estimation, Reconstruction & Analysis

3.1 Motivation and Clinical Applications 34

3.2 Acquisition and Contrast Protocol 35

3.3 Motion Estimation and Compensation via Surface Model 35

3.4 Ventricle Motion Analysis 43

3.5 Evaluation and Results 46

3.6 Challenges. 72

3.7 Summary and Conclusions 73

In clinical practice, when patients undergo a coronary examination, the function and morphology of the left ventricle (LV) is investigated [Krak 04]. The analysis of the ventriculogram is usually done to visualize and quantify the ventricular function. The quantification in the catheter lab is based on the temporal sequence of 2-D X-ray images, but no 3-D+t volumetric information is provided. A C-arm system provides the possibility to acquire rotational angiographic 2-D projection images from different views. These projections can be used for 3-D imaging. The image acquisition using a C-arm CT system requires several seconds. A standard FDK reconstruction using all acquired projection images results in a motion blurred image. One possibility to improve temporal resolution, is the retrospective ECG-gating from a single C-arm rotation as described in Section 2.3.1. However, a retrospective ECG-gated tomographic reconstruction suffers from severe undersampling artifacts. These artifacts occur from the fact that a single scan with an acquisition time of 5 s to 8 s covers only 5 to 10 cardiac cycles. Therefore, novel motion estimation and compensation techniques are required.

This chapter describes a surface-based motion estimation, reconstruction and analysis framework for the LV in the catheter laboratory using a C-arm device. First, the motivation and the clinical application are described in more detail in Section 3.1. The exact acquisition and contrast protocol of the C-arm CT scan are described in Section 3.2. In Section 3.3, the generation of the dynamic surface mesh is presented. As the 3-D motion compensation requires a dense motion vector field, the sparse motion vector field defined only at the LV surface needs to be mapped to a dense

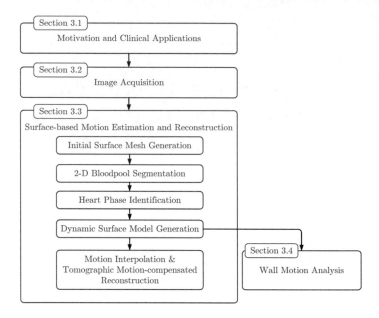

Figure 3.1: Schematic overview of the surface-based motion estimation, reconstruction and analysis.

motion vector field (MVF), cf. Section 2.5.2. Different interpolation schemes were evaluated with respect to the reconstruction quality and accuracy.

Furthermore, the surface model provides also the possibility to analyze the wall motion of the LV, presented in Section 3.4. Different parameters to extract motion defects like dyssynchrony information of the LV ventricle are transferred from different modalities to use them for wall motion analysis in combination with a C-arm CT. The results of the interpolation techniques to compute dense MVFs and the wall motion analysis parameter are presented in Section 3.5. The second to last section, Section 3.6 discusses the challenges of the presented methods and Section 3.7 summarizes this chapter. A schematic overview of the surface-based motion estimation, reconstruction and analysis is given in Figure 3.1.

Parts of this work have already been published in Chen et al. [Chen 11, Chen 13c], and Müller et al. [Mlle 12b, Mlle 13c, Mlle 13b, Mlle 14c].

3.1   Motivation and Clinical Applications

In interventional procedures, there is increasing interest in four-dimensional imaging of dynamic cardiac shapes, e.g., the left ventricle (LV), for quantitative evaluation of cardiac functions such as ejection fraction and wall motion analysis. An angiographic C-arm CT system is capable of acquiring multiple 2-D projections while rotating around the patient. With such data a 3-D reconstruction of the imaged region is possible. Due to the long acquisition time, a few seconds, of the C-arm, imaging of dynamic structures presents a challenge. The motion of the heart ventricle needs to be taken into account in the reconstruction process. The standard FDK algorithm [Feld 84] as presented in Section 2.2.1 would use all acquired projections for reconstruction. Consequently, different heart phases cannot be distinguished. The result would be a motion blurred reconstruction of the heart ventricle. A motion-compensated tomographic reconstruction for the heart ventricle could overcome the limitations of the FDK approach. In order to compensate for the motion [Schf 06], the dynamics of the heart need to be estimated.

Up to now, no quantitative 3-D/4-D analysis of the left ventricle (LV) has been performed during the intervention using angiographic C-arm CT. Functional information is provided by other devices, mainly ultrasound (US) [Kape 05, Jenk 04], magnetic resonance imaging (MRI) [Matt 12, Ma 12] or cardiac computed tomography angiography (CCTA) [Lee 12, Po 11]. The three-dimensional echocardiography, CCTA and MRI have to be performed before the cardiac intervention. In this chapter, the goal is a one-step solution of functional cardiac imaging directly inside the catheter lab with the interventional C-arm system, since C-arm systems are the main modality used for performing fluoroscopic imaging. A combination of a motion-compensated reconstruction with a quantitative analysis of the dynamics of the left heart ventricle (LV) would provide a cardiologist with valuable diagnostic information. The LV motion information could also improve the outcome of complex cardiac procedures, such as cardiac resynchronization therapy (CRT) [De B 13a]. The LV model can guide a physician to an optimal position of the LV lead and hence, increase the rate of success of these interventions [Ma 12].

3.2   Acquisition and Contrast Protocol

The image acquisition protocol for an LV scan with a C-arm system consists of a few hundred projection images over an angular range of $200°$ in $5\,\mathrm{s}$ to $8\,\mathrm{s}$ during a breath hold. Contrast agent is administered directly into the LV via a pigtail catheter inserted through the femoral artery in the leg or radial/brachial artery in the arm. Imaging starts with a delay of about $1\,\mathrm{s}$, the time required for the contrast to fill the LV homogeneously.

The porcine dataset was acquired in a research laboratory at Stanford University and the clinical datasets were provided by the Universitätsklinikum Erlangen and the Thoraxcenter, Erasmus MC Rotterdam.

3.3   Motion Estimation and Compensation via Surface Model

The individual steps in order to compute a dynamic surface model of the LV and to use it for motion-compensated reconstruction, are the following: (1) fitting an initial mesh to the standard FDK reconstruction [Feld 84] using all projection images, (2) segmentation of the 2-D bloodpool, (3) heart phase identification, (4) adaptation of the surface mesh, (5) dense MVF motion estimation from generated surface model, (6) limitation of the motion to a region of interest, and (7) motion-compensated tomographic reconstruction. The individual steps are explained in more detail in the following subsections.

3.3.1   Initial Surface Mesh Generation

As initialization, a standard FDK reconstruction is performed using all available 2-D projections. This reconstruction exhibits artifacts due to cardiac motion, but the reconstruction quality is sufficient for extraction of a static and preliminary 3-D LV endocardium mesh using a marginal space learning and steerable feature approach proposed by Zheng et al. [Zhen 08].

3.3.2   2-D Bloodpool Segmentation

The 2-D bloodpool segmentation is based on a boundary defined by a set of connected points. For each of these points, the steerable features [Zhen 08] centered at this point location are extracted to train a probabilistic boosting tree (PBT) classifier [Tu 05]. During the training stage, the manually annotated LV bloodpool boundary is given as the input to extract positive samples (on the true boundary) and negative samples (far away from the boundary). During testing, the initial generated surface mesh is forward projected onto the 2-D projection images and the contour of the forward projected mesh is detected [Chen 11]. Features along the normal direction of the contour are extracted as the input to the trained classifier, and the candidate location with the peak probability score is selected as detected contour location [Chen 11]. The bloodpool segmentation results in the 2-D bloodpool size signal $\pi(i) \in \mathbb{Z}^+$ given in pixels.

3.3.3   Heart Phase Identification

The heart phase $\phi(i) \in [0, 1]$ of each projection image needs to be identified. For patients with an irregular heart rhythm the cardiac phase cannot be assigned from the electrocardiogram (ECG) signal by linear interpolation between two R-R peaks in the same manner as with a regular heart beat [Laur 06]. Therefore, the 2-D segmented bloodpool area is used for identification of the heart phase. The 2-D bloodpool size $\pi(i) \in \mathbb{Z}^+$ at acquisition angle i, given as the segmented area in pixels in the 2-D projection images is filtered with a 1-D Gaussian kernel in order to obtain a smoothed bloodpool curve $\pi_f(i)$, cf. Figure 3.2a. The minimum and maximum points are then identified as candidate points for end-systole (ES) i_{ES} and end-diastole (ED) i_{ED}. A pre-defined threshold is used to exclude false local maxima and minima, cf. Figure 3.2a, frames 102 and 110. The detected ED's divide the signal $\pi_f(i)$ into multiple cardiac cycles. In order to generate a reference time-size curve $\overline{\pi}(\xi)$, an intermediate heart phase $\xi \in [0, 1]$ is introduced

$$\xi = \frac{i - i_{ED1}}{i_{ED2} - i_{ED1}}, \tag{3.1}$$

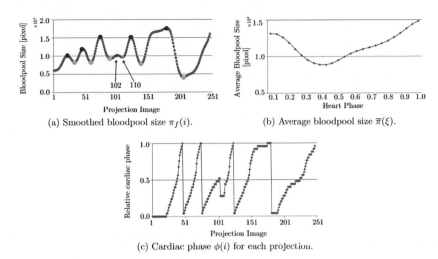

(a) Smoothed bloodpool size $\pi_f(i)$.   (b) Average bloodpool size $\overline{\pi}(\xi)$.

(c) Cardiac phase $\phi(i)$ for each projection.

Figure 3.2: Examples of (a) a smoothed bloodpool segmentation size $\pi_f(i)$ and (b) the mean bloodpool signal $\overline{\pi}(\xi)$ by averaging multiple cardiac cycles. (c) shows the derived cardiac phase $\phi(i)$ based on Equation (3.4). The candidate end-diastole (ED) time i_{ED} and end-systole (ES) time i_{ES} are marked as red and green dots and the red and green ring mark the additional smaller contraction in (a).

where i_{ED1} and i_{ED2} are the first and last ED point of the current cycle. The bloodpool curve of each cycle is temporally re-sampled to fit to an average length of a cardiac cycle. The re-sampled curves are then averaged over all cycles to generate $\overline{\pi}(\xi)$. An example of a reference curve $\overline{\pi}(\xi)$ is shown in Figure 3.2b. In order to eliminate the size variation of the bloodpool due to the rotation of the C-arm system, a normalized bloodpool size $\pi_n(i)$ is computed as follows:

$$\pi_n(i) = \begin{cases} \frac{\pi_f(i)-\pi_f(i_{ES})}{\pi_f(i_{ED1})-\pi_f(i_{ES})} \cdot (\overline{\pi}(0) - \overline{\pi}(\xi_{ES})) + \overline{\pi}(\xi_{ES}), & i < i_{ES} \\ \frac{\pi_f(i)-\pi_f(i_{ES})}{\pi_f(i_{ED2})-\pi_f(i_{ES})} \cdot (\overline{\pi}(1) - \overline{\pi}(\xi_{ES})) + \overline{\pi}(\xi_{ES}), & i \geq i_{ES} \end{cases}, \qquad (3.2)$$

where ξ_{ES} is the ES time point of the reference curve $\overline{\pi}(\xi)$, with

$$\xi_{ES} = \arg\min_{\xi} \overline{\pi}(\xi) \qquad (3.3)$$

and i_{ES} is the end-systolic point of the cardiac cycle containing the currently considered frame. Finally, the cardiac phase $\phi(i)$ for each projection and time point can be obtained based on a quasi-inverse mapping of $\overline{\pi}(\xi)$ at the systolic and diastolic period separately,

$$\phi(i) = \overline{\pi}^{-1}(\pi_n(i)), \qquad (3.4)$$

where a systolic period is present if $i < i_{ES}$ and a diastolic period otherwise. The continuous heart phase $\phi(i)$ is binned into a number of K heart phases by nearest-neighbor classification and denoted with ϕ_k, with $k = 1, \ldots, K$. The number of heart phases K can be chosen according to the number of frames per heart cycle. An example of a derived cardiac phase signal $\phi(i)$ is given in Figure 3.2c. If a local maximum is detected which is not ED, as illustrated in Figure 3.2a at frame 102, the phase labeling process based on Equation (3.4) is reset to the systolic period. At the beginning and end of the scan, if no full cardiac cycle is detected, the local maximum and minimum are used for fitting the half cycle to the average bloodpool signal and the cardiac phase can be assigned as previously described. In the example shown in Figure 3.2a no local minimum is detected at the beginning and hence the heart phases at the beginning of the scan are set to zero, as depicted in Figure 3.2c.

3.3.4   Dynamic Surface Model Generation

The proposed motion-compensated reconstruction uses a motion vector field (MVF) estimate given by a dynamic 3-D surface model of the ventricle generated from the 2-D projection data [Chen 11]. The projections are assigned to certain heart phases corresponding to the bloodpool size signal generated from the 2-D projection images described in Section 3.3.3. The static mesh is then projected onto the 2-D projections belonging to a certain heart phase. The projected mesh silhouette is adjusted in the direction of the normal to each control point in order to match the 2-D ventricle bloodpool border, cf. Section 3.3.2. The 2-D deformation vector is then transformed into the 3-D space and the 3-D mesh is updated accordingly. As a result a 3-D mesh is generated for every heart phase ϕ_k with its control points $\boldsymbol{p}_c(\phi_k) \in \mathbb{R}^3$, with $c = 1, \ldots, P_c$, where P_c is the number of control points [Chen 11].

For reconstruction, a reference heart phase ϕ_r is selected. The displacement or motion vectors point in the direction of the motion of the sparse control points between different heart phases. They are denoted as $\boldsymbol{d}_c(\phi_k) \in \mathbb{R}^3$ describing the distance of every control point between the reference heart phase ϕ_r and the current heart phase ϕ_k. They can then be computed by

$$\boldsymbol{d}_c(\phi_k) = \boldsymbol{p}_c(\phi_k) - \boldsymbol{p}_c(\phi_r). \tag{3.5}$$

An example of the left ventricle surface model for two different heart phases at end-diastole and end-systole is illustrated in Figure 3.3a. In Figure 3.3b, the sparse motion vectors $\boldsymbol{d}_c(\phi_k)$ are shown between the reference heart phase and the current heart phase.

3.3.5   Different Motion Interpolation Techniques

In order to perform a motion-compensated tomographic reconstruction as described in Section 2.5.2, a dense motion vector field (MVF) needs to be generated from the sparse MVF. For every projection image i the assignment to a heart phase ϕ_k is known, cf. Section 3.3.3. The motion model function $M : \mathbb{N} \times \mathbb{R}^3 \times \mathbb{R}^{K_{\mathrm{mm}}} \mapsto \mathbb{R}^3$ describes the mapping from a reference phase ϕ_r to the current heart phase ϕ_k and is described by

$$M(\phi_k, \boldsymbol{x}, \tilde{\boldsymbol{s}}_{\mathrm{mm}}) = \boldsymbol{x} + \boldsymbol{d}(\boldsymbol{x}, \tilde{\boldsymbol{s}}_{\mathrm{mm}}), \tag{3.6}$$

where $\boldsymbol{d}(\boldsymbol{x}, \tilde{\boldsymbol{s}}_{\mathrm{mm}}) \in \mathbb{R}^3$ denotes the displacement vector at voxel position $\boldsymbol{x}$ and $\tilde{\boldsymbol{s}}_{\mathrm{mm}} \in \mathbb{R}^{\widetilde{K}_{\mathrm{mm}}}$ the motion vector parameters between reference and current heart phase. In

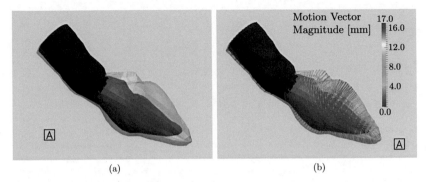

Figure 3.3: Illustration of the extracted surface model of the left ventricle. (a) Surface model for two different heart phases at end-diastole (transparent) and end-systole (solid). (b) Sparse motion vectors $d_c(\phi_k)$ between reference heart phase at end-diastole (transparent) and current phase at end-systole (solid).

order to result in a complete definition of the cardiac motion over the whole scan, the motion needs to be estimated between the reference heart phase ϕ_r and all remaining $K - 1$ heart phases. Different interpolation methods to provide the displacement vectors were evaluated and are explained below.

3.3.5.1 Thin-Plate Splines (TPS)

The deformation of the LV between two time points can be represented by a thin-plate spline (TPS) transformation. The TPS approach assumes that the bending and stretching behavior of the left ventricle is similar to the bending of a thin plate. Thin-plate splines have already been applied to estimate cardiac vascular motion for CT data [Isol 10b] and ventricular motion for MRI data [Sute 00]. Furthermore, they are widely used for elastic image registration of medical images [Spre 96, Rohr 01].

For describing a transformation by a thin-plate spline between two heart phases, $\widetilde{K}_{\mathrm{mm}} = (3 \cdot (3P_c) + 9 + 3) = 3 \cdot (3P_c) + 12$ parameters are required, i.e. $\tilde{s}_{\mathrm{mm}} = (p(\phi_r), p(\phi_k), c(\phi_k), a(\phi_k), b(\phi_k))^T$, where $p(\phi_r) \in \mathbb{R}^{3P_c}$, $p(\phi_k) \in \mathbb{R}^{3P_c}$ are a linearized version of the surface control points at the current and the reference heart phase. The vector $c(\phi_k) \in \mathbb{R}^{3P_c}$ is also a linearized version of the spline coefficients of $c_c(\phi_k) \in \mathbb{R}^3$ for each control point, with $c = 1, \ldots, P_c$. The vector $a(\phi_k) \in \mathbb{R}^9$ contains the linearized rotation, shearing, and scaling parameters of an affine transformation matrix $A(\phi_k) \in \mathbb{R}^{3 \times 3}$. The parameter $b(\phi_k) \in \mathbb{R}^3$ is a translation vector. The TPS coordinate transformation with its displacements for an arbitrary point $x \in \mathbb{R}^3$ is then given as

$$d(x, \tilde{s}_{\mathrm{mm}}) \;=\; \sum_{c=1}^{P_c} G(x - p_c(\phi_k))c_c(\phi_k) + A(\phi_k)x + b(\phi_k), \qquad (3.7)$$

where $\boldsymbol{d}(\boldsymbol{x}, \tilde{\boldsymbol{s}}_{\mathrm{mm}})$ is the displacement vector at point $\boldsymbol{x}$ and $\boldsymbol{p}_c(\phi_k) \in \mathbb{R}^3$ is one control point. The transformation's kernel matrix $\boldsymbol{G}(\boldsymbol{x}) \in \mathbb{R}^{3 \times 3}$ of a point $\boldsymbol{x} \in \mathbb{R}^3$ for a 3-D TPS is given according to [Davi 97]

$$\boldsymbol{G}(\boldsymbol{x}) = r(\boldsymbol{x}) \cdot \boldsymbol{I}, \tag{3.8}$$
$$r(\boldsymbol{x}) = ||\boldsymbol{x}||_2, \tag{3.9}$$

where $\boldsymbol{I} \in \mathbb{R}^{3 \times 3}$ is the identity matrix. In order to solve Equation (3.7) for each ϕ_k, set $\boldsymbol{d}(\boldsymbol{x}, \tilde{\boldsymbol{s}}_{\mathrm{mm}}) = \boldsymbol{d}_c(\phi_k)$ for $\boldsymbol{x} = \boldsymbol{p}_c(\phi_k)$. Farther away from the control points, the distance from the point to all control points is quite large. Hence the first part of Equation (3.7) becomes a multiple of the average of $\boldsymbol{c}_c(\phi_k)$ and is reduced to an affine transformation. As Equation (3.7) is linear in $\boldsymbol{c}_c(\phi_k)$, $\boldsymbol{A}(\phi_k)$, and $\boldsymbol{b}(\phi_k)$, it can be solved in a straightforward manner [Davi 97].

The resulting spline coefficients and affine parameters are inserted in Equation (3.7) in order to evaluate the spline at any arbitrary 3-D point. A motion vector can therefore be computed for every voxel in the reconstructed volume. In order to find a complete cardiac motion over the whole scan, the motion needs to be estimated between the reference heart phase ϕ_r and the remaining $K-1$ heart phases. Therefore, the dimension of the motion vector parameter for all heart phases is $\boldsymbol{s}_{\mathrm{mm}} \in \mathbb{R}^{K_{\mathrm{mm}}}$ with $K_{\mathrm{mm}} = (K - 1) \cdot (3 \cdot 3P_c + 12)$.

3.3.5.2 Linear Interpolation

For linear interpolation, surface control points around the point $\boldsymbol{x}$ are determined and the resulting displacement vector $\boldsymbol{d}(\boldsymbol{x}, \tilde{\boldsymbol{s}}_{\mathrm{mm}})$ is a weighted sum of the corresponding displacement vectors

$$\boldsymbol{d}(\boldsymbol{x}, \tilde{\boldsymbol{s}}_{\mathrm{mm}}) = \sum_{c=1}^{P_c} \boldsymbol{G}^*(\boldsymbol{x} - \boldsymbol{p}_c(\phi_k)) \boldsymbol{d}_c(\phi_k), \tag{3.10}$$
$$\boldsymbol{G}^*(\boldsymbol{x}) = u(\boldsymbol{x}) \cdot \boldsymbol{I}, \tag{3.11}$$

where u is a weighting function. Function u weights the displacement vectors according to the distance between the control point $\boldsymbol{p}_c(\phi_k)$ and the point $\boldsymbol{x}$. Three weighting functions were investigated. For describing a transformation by a linear interpolation between two heart phases, $\widehat{K}_{\mathrm{mm}} = 2 \cdot 3P_c + 1$ parameters are required, i.e. $\tilde{\boldsymbol{s}}_{\mathrm{mm}} = (\boldsymbol{p}(\phi_r), \boldsymbol{p}(\phi_k), l)^T$, where $l \in \mathbb{N}$ can be a number of points n_c used for interpolation or $l \in \mathbb{R}$ can be a radius R defining a region in which points contribute to the linear interpolation. The motion vectors $\boldsymbol{d}(\phi_k)$ are a linearized version of $\boldsymbol{d}_c(\phi_k)$ and are defined by Equation (3.5). In order to result in a complete cardiac motion over the whole scan, the motion needs to be estimated between the reference heart phase ϕ_r and the remaining $K-1$ heart phases. Therefore, the dimension of the motion vector parameter for all heart phases is $\boldsymbol{s}_{\mathrm{mm}} \in \mathbb{R}^{K_{\mathrm{mm}}}$ with $K_{\mathrm{mm}} = (K - 1) \cdot (2 \cdot 3P_c + 1)$.

Shepard's Method. An inverse distance weighting is applied according to the distance from the considered point to the n_c closest control points [Shep 68]. The function u is therefore defined as

$$u(\boldsymbol{x}) = \frac{||\boldsymbol{x}||_2^{-1}}{\sum_{j=1}^{n_c} || (\boldsymbol{x} - \boldsymbol{p}_j(\phi_k)) ||_2^{-1}}. \tag{3.12}$$

Smoothed Weighting Function. In this case, the function u is a cosine-based smoothing function

$$u(\boldsymbol{x}) = \begin{cases} \frac{1}{\mathcal{W}}(1 + \cos(\frac{\|\boldsymbol{x}\|_2 \cdot \pi}{R})) & , \text{ if } \|\boldsymbol{x}\|_2 \leq R \\ 0 & \text{ otherwise,} \end{cases} \tag{3.13}$$

where $\mathcal{W}$ denotes a normalization constant so that $\sum_{j=1}^{W_c} u(\boldsymbol{x}_j) = 1$, and $\boldsymbol{x}_j = \boldsymbol{x} - \boldsymbol{p}_j(\phi_k)$. The number of points inside the radius R is given by W_c.

Simple Averaging. Here the resulting displacement vector $\boldsymbol{d}(\boldsymbol{x}, \tilde{\boldsymbol{s}}_{\mathrm{mm}})$ is a simple average of the displacement vectors at the surrounding control points. Thus, the function u, with W_c denoting the number of control points located within a sphere of radius R around $\boldsymbol{x}$ is defined as

$$u(\boldsymbol{x}) = \begin{cases} \frac{1}{W_c} & , \text{ if } \|\boldsymbol{x}\|_2 \leq R \\ 0 & \text{ otherwise.} \end{cases} \tag{3.14}$$

3.3.6 Cutting

In order to reduce the computational complexity, it is assumed that the left ventricle is the central moving organ inside the scan field of view. This assumption is justified due to the acquisition protocol where - for the most part - only the left heart ventricle is filled with contrast during the procedure. Therefore, a dense MVF is estimated in the neighborhood of the ventricle. The considered set of points $\mathcal{P}$, for which a motion vector is estimated, is given as

$$\mathcal{P} = \{\boldsymbol{x} \mid \|\boldsymbol{x} - \boldsymbol{p}_x(\phi_k)\|_2 \leq r_c\}, \tag{3.15}$$

where $\boldsymbol{p}_x(\phi_k)$ is the closest surface control point to the current point $\boldsymbol{x}$. In Figure 3.4a, an MVF of a human dataset between the reference heart phase at end-diastole and the current heart phase at end-systole is illustrated for the TPS. The MVF between the reference heart phase close to end-diastole and the current heart phase at end-diastole is illustrated for the TPS in Figure 3.4b.

3.3.7 Motion-Compensated Reconstruction

The motion-compensated reconstruction algorithm used here is based on the FDK formulation as described in Section 2.5.2.2. For every projection image i the assignment to a heart phase ϕ_k is known, cf. Section 3.3.3. Therefore, the estimated motion vector fields $M(i, \boldsymbol{x}, \boldsymbol{s}_{\mathrm{mm}})$ can be incorporated into a voxel-driven filtered backprojection reconstruction algorithm. The motion correction is applied during the backprojection step by shifting the voxel $\boldsymbol{x}$ to be reconstructed according to the motion vector function M. A more detailed explanation of the algorithm is provided in Section 2.5.2 of this thesis.

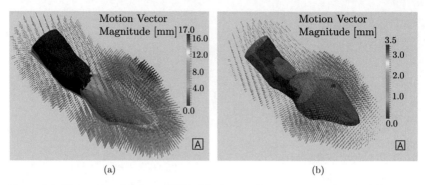

(a)   (b)

Figure 3.4: Illustration of a dense MVF of the human dataset computed with TPS around $r = 2$ cm of the LV surface. (a) Dense MVF between reference heart phase at end-diastole and current phase at end-systole. (b) Dense MVF between reference heart phase close to end-diastole and current phase at end-diastole. The number of vectors displayed has been reduced in order to permit visualization of MVF characteristics.

3.3.8   Complexity Analysis

In order to analyze the complexity of the different motion interpolation schemes, the $\mathcal{O}$-calculus is given for each method. For the thin-plate spline approach, the most complex part is to solve the linear equation system, e.g., with a singular value decomposition (SVD). The complexity of the SVD is dependent on the dimension of the matrix to be decomposed. Here, the matrix L has a dimension of $(3P_c + 12) \times (3P_c + 12)$ and increases with the number of the surface control points [Davi 97]. Therefore, the complexity results in $\mathcal{O}((3P_c + 12)^3)$, since all matrices U, Σ, V^T of the decomposition of L are required [Golu 96]. For the linear methods, the complexity scales linearly with the number of surface control points P_c, which results in $\mathcal{O}(P_c)$. All interpolation techniques scale with the number of heart phases ϕ_k. A number of $K - 1$ need to be computed in order to estimate all deformations.

Additionally, all techniques are used for a motion-compensated filtered-backprojection reconstruction. Given the side length of the 3-D volume n and the number of projections N, the complexity of a backprojection-based reconstruction is expressed as $\mathcal{O}(N\,n^3)$.

3.3.9   Implementation Details and Parameter Setting

In order to estimate a dense motion vector field, the various approaches have different parameters to be set. The thin-plate spline approach has only one parameter to adjust, the stiffness. This parameter defines whether the splines need to pass through the control points exactly or whether a given relaxation is allowed. The stiffness was set to 0 in all experiments carried out, i.e. no relaxation was allowed. For computation of the spline coefficients and the affine transformation parameters, a singular value decomposition (SVD) was used to solve the linear equation system in Equation (3.7).

This part was implemented in a straightforward manner on the CPU and is a critical point with respect to computational complexity, see Section 3.3.8. In order to speed up the runtime, the TPS transformation of each voxel was computed on the graphics card using CUDA [Sand 10] in order to take advantage of the parallelism of modern hardware.

For the linear extrapolation methods, different parameters need to be defined. For the Shepard's method, a certain number of considered neighboring points needs to be given. In this thesis, this number n_c was empirically set to 30. Due to the density of the grid points, the number $n_c = 30$ (total number of surface points 545) corresponds to a range of approximately 2 cm around each voxel x. Forthmann et al. [Fort 08] evaluated $n_c = 1$ and $n_c = 128$ neighbors and stated that the number of points can be selected to be quite small, but one neighbor point may not be sufficient. Regarding the smoothed weighting function and the simple averaging, a radius R is configured, here R is heuristically set to 2 cm. The region of interest distance r_c was heuristically set to 2 cm around the LV surface model in the heart phase ϕ_r.

The motion-compensated FDK reconstruction is also implemented on the GPU based on the work of [Sche 11, Wein 08].

3.4   Ventricle Motion Analysis

In the previous sections, the surface model was used to compute a tomographic motion-compensated reconstruction of different heart phases. In this section, the LV surface is used to analyze the contraction behavior of the LV with respect to pathological regions. First, the local coordinate system of the LV is introduced. The motion analysis part is divided into the volumetric computation of the LV, wall motion analysis in 3-D and a mapping of the 3-D motion information to an overview map in 2-D. The individual steps are explained in more detail in the following sections.

The wall motion analysis software was implemented on the CPU and is operated via a graphical user interface implemented with the Qt Project[1] and the visualization of the surface meshes is based on the Visualization Toolkit[2] (vtk) [Schr 06].

3.4.1   Left Ventricle Representation

In order to analyze the contraction behavior of the LV, an orthogonal local coordinate system is introduced. The three orthogonal main axes of the end-diastolic LV surface are computed by a modified principal component analysis (PCA) with a rotation and an adjustment of the centroid. The coordinate system is kept fixed for the whole analysis. The first principal axis $n_1 \in \mathbb{R}^3$ points towards the long axis of the LV between the apex point and the middle point of the mitral valve. The second axis $n_2 \in \mathbb{R}^3$, points into the anterior direction and the third axis $n_3 \in \mathbb{R}^3$ in the septal direction. Initially, n_1 does not necessarily pass through the apex, since the LV is not necessarily symmetric. Therefore, the coordinate system (n_1, n_2, n_3) is rotated to align n_1 with the long axis. The origin of the coordinate system is defined as the mid

---

[1]http://qt-project.org/
[2]http://www.vtk.org/

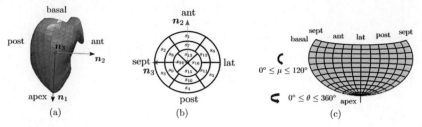

Figure 3.5: (a) Septal view of one left ventricle surface model at end-diastole with the local coordinate system (n_1, n_2, n_3). n_3 is pointing towards the reader. (b) Circumferential polar plot of the 16 myocardial segments with the used coordinate system (n_1, n_2, n_3). n_1 is pointing towards the reader. Image according to [Cerq 02]. (c) Hammer projection used to preserve the areas while mapping varying measures of function from 3-D to 2-D. Image according to [Herz 05].

point between base and apex. A schematic of the three coordinate axes is provided in Figure 3.5a.

The LV surface is divided into 16 segments according to the recommendation of the American Heart Association (AHA) for the myocardium and each point p_c is assigned to one of these segments [Cerq 02]. The 16 myocardial segments are illustrated in Figure 3.5b.

3.4.2 Motion Analysis

In order to provide a broad portfolio of functional parameters to the cardiologist, a wall motion analysis is performed in 3-D as well as a mapping of the 3-D motion information to a overview map in 2-D called Hammer projection.

3.4.2.1 Volume Computation

For every heart phase the three-dimensional LV volume $\Pi(i) \in \mathbb{R}^+$ is computed. The mapping between the heart phase and each acquisition time point i is known, cf. Section 3.3.3. The end-diastolic volume (EDV) and end-systolic volume (ESV) are determined as maximum and minimum volume. The ejection fraction (EF) is the difference between the end-diastolic volume and the end-systolic volume compared to the end-diastolic volume. The EF is computed as

$$\mathrm{EF}[\%] = \frac{\mathrm{EDV\text{-}ESV}}{\mathrm{EDV}} . \qquad (3.16)$$

A normal EF has a lower limit of about 50 %, below that value the contraction ability of the LV is impaired [Pfis 85].

3.4.2.2   Wall Motion in 3-D

The ventricular wall motion can be analyzed in 3-D using different features adapted from other modalities (CCTA, US, MR):

Heart Phase to Maximal Contraction ($\phi_{c,\mathbf{max}}$).   The minimal Euclidean distance $\lambda_c(\phi_k)$ from every point $\boldsymbol{p}_c(\phi_k)$ to the long axis $\boldsymbol{n}_1$ can be computed. In order to eliminate small outliers, the distance signals are temporally filtered by a mean filter with a kernel size of 5. Finally, for every surface point, the phase until it reaches its maximum of contraction $\phi_{c,\mathrm{max}}$ can be determined. For synchronous LV motion, a uniform distribution over the entire LV surface can be observed. A higher variability in the contraction times occurs for dyssynchronous dynamics [Po 11].

Systolic Dyssynchrony Index (SDI).   The systolic dyssynchrony index (SDI) known from echocardiography [Gime 08, Kape 05, Sach 11] can be estimated with the LV volumetric information for every heart phase. For each surface point $\boldsymbol{p}_c(\phi_k)$ the associated myocardial segment is known and fixed for all heart phases. Therefore, the subvolume of each segment can be determined by dividing the LV surface into small triangle pyramids given by the surface mesh and the mid point of the LV mesh points. In order to eliminate small outliers, the subvolume signals are temporally filtered by a mean filter with a kernel size of 5. For each segment, the phase $\phi_{s,\mathrm{max}}$ of maximal contraction and the overall mean phase of maximal contraction ϕ_{max} for all segments are computed. The standard deviation of the maximal contraction phases between the segments is an indicator for LV synchrony

$$\mathrm{SDI} = \sqrt{\frac{1}{16}\sum_{s=1}^{16}(\phi_{s,\mathrm{max}} - \phi_{\mathrm{max}})^2}. \tag{3.17}$$

Since the SDI represents the standard deviation between contraction phases, a higher SDI denotes increased ventricular dyssynchrony. For echocardiography, Kapetanakis et al. stated an SDI $\leq$ 3.5±1.8 % as normal and mild disease for an SDI of 5.4±0.8 %, moderate disease for an SDI of 10.0±2 % and a severe disease for an SDI of 15.6±1 % [Kape 05]. It should be mentioned that the SDI is a relatively new parameter of dyssynchrony and there is still variation between the methods of measurement [Sach 11], but irrespective of the analysis software, there is an agreement that healthy individuals rarely have SDI values over 6%.

Three-dimensional Fractional Shortening (3DFS$_c$).   In 2-D echocardiography, the fractional shortening of the LV is used as an indicator to identify pathological dynamics. Ischemic regions can be distinguished from normal areas of the LV. It specifies the relationship between the LV radius in diastole and its decrease during systole. Here, a three-dimensional fractional shortening (3DFS$_c$) can be computed similar to [Herz 05]. The 3DFS$_c$ value for every point is defined as

$$3\mathrm{DFS}_c = \frac{\lambda_{c,\mathrm{ED}} - \lambda_{c,\mathrm{ES}}}{\lambda_{c,\mathrm{ED}}}, \tag{3.18}$$

where $\lambda_{c,\text{ED}}$ and $\lambda_{c,\text{ES}}$ denote the Euclidean distance of the mesh point $\boldsymbol{p}_c(\phi_k)$ to the long axis $\boldsymbol{n}_1$ in end-diastole and end-systole, respectively. Herz et al. classified the wall motion as normal ($3\text{DFS}_c > 0.25$), hypokinetic ($0.05 < 3\text{DFS}_c \leq 0.25$), akinetic ($-0.05 < 3\text{DFS}_c \leq 0.05$) or dyskinetic ($3\text{DFS}_c \leq -0.05$). The lower limit of normal is based on the standards for 2-D fractional shortening of the American Society of Echocardiography while the values to separate akinesis and dyskinesis are chosen arbitrarily [Herz 05].

3.4.2.3 Hammer Projection

In order to provide the point-based indicators in an overview map, a Hammer projection map is created [Hunt 88]. The maximal contraction phase $\phi_{c,\text{max}}$ and the fractional shortening 3DFS_c are mapped from the LV mesh surface to 2-D as a function of location from apex to base ($0° \leq \mu \leq 120°$) and circumferential position ($0° < \theta \leq 360°$). The Hammer projection maps the surface motion information to 2-D while preserving relative surface areas, cf. Figure 3.5c [Hunt 88]. The LV surface is represented by a small number of control points, therefore, the surface with its point-based motion information is re-sampled. The surface is re-sampled with an angular increment of $0.25°$ degrees in the μ and θ directions. The scalar value at the sample point is computed by simple averaging of the information given at the neighboring triangle vertices ($\phi_{c,\text{max}}$ or 3DFS_c).

3.5   Evaluation and Results

In the following sections, the evaluation of the motion estimation and compensation algorithm and ventricular wall motion analysis is presented. The motion estimation and compensation part was evaluated on a generated phantom dataset as well as on a porcine model and on three real clinical patient datasets. The wall motion analysis was performed on specifically designed phantoms with pathological contraction behavior and eight clinical datasets in total. Among them were two patient datasets, which were also evaluated for the motion estimation and compensation algorithm.

3.5.1   Motion Estimation and Reconstruction

In order to evaluate the interpolation scheme of the motion estimation and reconstruction algorithm, the reconstruction quality of the phantom data was evaluated with respect to the 3-D reconstruction quality of the image compared to a gold standard reconstruction. Furthermore, the phantom data as well as the clinical datasets were analyzed regarding the accuracy of the forward projection of the motion-compensated reconstructions compared to the 2-D LV bloodpool boundary.

3.5.1.1   Datasets

Three different kinds of datasets were used for motion estimation and compensation evaluation, one phantom, one porcine and three clinical patient datasets.

Ventricular Phantom.   The algorithm presented here has been applied to a ventricle dataset comparable to the XCAT phantom [Sega 08, Maie 12, Maie 13]. The bloodpool density of the left ventricle was set to $2.5\,\text{g/cm}^3$, the density of the myocardium wall to $1.5\,\text{g/cm}^3$ and the blood in the aorta to $2.0\,\text{g/cm}^3$. It is assumed that all materials have the same absorption as water. Data was simulated using a clinical protocol with the following parameters: 395 projection images simulated equi-angularly over an angular range of about $200°$ degrees with an angular increment of $0.5°/\text{f}$ at a frame rate of 60 fps with a size of 620×480 pixels at an isotropic resolution of $0.62\,\text{mm/pixel}$ and a scan time of about 8 s. The distance from source to detector was 120 cm and from source to isocenter 78 cm, leading to a resolution of about 0.4 mm in the isocenter. The surface model consisted of $K = 40$ heart phases between subsequent R-peaks and $P_c = 957$ control points uniformly distributed over the left ventricle. The image reconstruction was performed on an image volume of $(25.6\,\text{cm})^3$ distributed on a 256^3 voxel grid. Physiological parameters extracted from the surface model p_0 are given in Table 3.1.

Porcine Model.   The porcine dataset was acquired on an Axiom Artis dTA C-arm system (Siemens AG, Healthcare Sector, Forchheim, Germany) at a research laboratory in Stanford. Data was acquired using the same clinical protocol as described in the paragraph above: 395 projection images sampled equi-angularly over an angular range of about $200°$ degrees with an angular increment of $0.5°/\text{f}$ at a frame rate of 60 fps with a size of 620×480 pixels at an isotropic resolution of $0.62\,\text{mm/pixel}$ and a scan time of about 8 s. The distance from source to detector was 120 cm and from source to isocenter 78 cm, leading to a resolution of about 0.4 mm in the isocenter. The undiluted contrast agent Omnipaque 350 (350 mg/ml) was administered at 15 ml/s via a pigtail catheter directly into the left heart ventricle, 1.5 s before the imaging started. The total injection time was 9.5 s and the pig had a weight of 62 kg. The surface model consisted of $K = 30$ heart phases between subsequent R-peaks and $P_c = 961$ control points equally distributed over the left ventricle. Image reconstruction was performed on an image volume of $(21.8\,\text{cm})^3$ distributed on a 256^3 voxel grid. Physiological parameters extracted from the surface model p_{por} are given in Table 3.1.

Clinical Data.   The first dataset h_1 was acquired on an Artis zee C-arm system (Siemens AG, Healthcare Sector, Forchheim, Germany) at the Thoraxcenter, Erasmus MC Rotterdam, Netherlands. It consists of 133 projection images acquired over an angular range of about $200°$ degrees with an angular increment of $1.5°/\text{f}$ in about 5 s with a size of 960×960 pixels at an isotropic resolution of $0.18\,\text{mm/pixel}$ (about 0.12 mm in isocenter) at a frame rate of 30 fps. The distance from source to detector was 120 cm and from source to isocenter 75 cm. The contrast agent was administered undiluted at 10 ml/s by a pigtail catheter directly into the left heart ventricle, with 1 s X-ray delay. The surface model consisted of $K = 26$ heart phases between subsequent R-peaks and $P_c = 961$ control points equally distributed over the first section of the aorta, outflow tract and left ventricle. Image reconstruction was performed on an image volume of $(14.1\,\text{cm})^3$ distributed on a 256^3 voxel grid.

	Heart rate [bpm]	EF [%]	SV [ml]	EDV [ml]	ESV [ml]
Phantom p_0	75	30.95	42.03	135.82	93.79
Porcine p_{por}	103.0 ± 24.2	45.80	40.05	87.44	47.40
Human h_1	61.6 ± 1.7	74.71	50.43	67.50	17.07
Human h_2	62.9 ± 2.9	58.73	65.14	110.91	45.77
Human h_3	55.3 ± 9.3	62.33	89.07	142.91	53.84

Table 3.1: Physiological data measurements of the motion estimation and compensation datasets extracted from the surface models: ejection fraction (EF), stroke volume (SV), end-diastolic volume (EDV), end-systolic volume (ESV).

The datasets h_2 and h_3 were acquired on an Artis zeego C-arm system (Siemens AG, Healthcare Sector, Forchheim, Germany) at the Thoraxcenter, Erasmus MC Rotterdam, Netherlands. They consist of 133 projection images acquired over an angular range of 200° with an angular increment of 1.5°/f in about 5 s with a size of 960×960 pixels at an isotropic resolution of 0.31 mm/pixel (about 0.2 mm in isocenter). The frame rate was 30 fps, the distance from source to detector was 120 cm and the distance from source to isocenter was 78 cm. The left heart ventricle was again filled with undiluted contrast directly by a pigtail catheter with 15 ml/s and 1 s X-ray delay. The surface model consisted of $K = 25$ and 30 heart phases between subsequent R-peaks for h_2 and h_3 respectively and 609 points equally distributed over the left ventricle and the outflow tract, and $P_c = 545$ control points define the left ventricle. Image reconstruction was performed on an image volume of $(19.2 \, \text{cm})^3$ distributed on a 256^3 voxel grid. Physiological parameters for h_1, h_2 and h_3 extracted from the surface models are given in Table 3.1.

3.5.1.2 Quantitative Evaluation Methods of 3-D Reconstruction Quality

For the phantom dataset, the accuracy of the motion-compensated reconstruction is also evaluated in the 3-D image space using the normalized root mean square error (nRMSE) and the universal image quality index (UQI). The deviation of the forward projection of the motion-compensated reconstructions and the left ventricular boundary in 2-D is analyzed for the phantom, the porcine and the three clinical datasets.

Phantom Image Quality in 3-D Image Space. For the dynamic phantom dataset the 3-D error and a quantitative 3-D image metric can be evaluated. In order to measure only the artifacts introduced by the heart motion, the FDK reconstruction of the static heart phantom of the same heart phase is used as gold standard. The ground truth of the phantom is not used due to the fact that only the artifacts coming from the heart motion should be measured and evaluated by using FDK as a gold standard. Other cone-beam or truncation artifacts are identical in the images and can be neglected. Heart phases from 10 % to 100 % with 10 % increment were evaluated. The reconstruction of the static phantom is done with the same

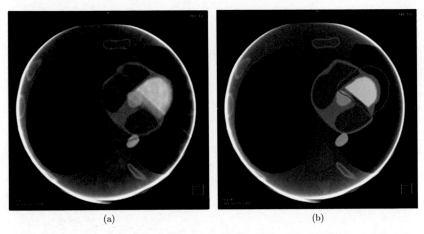

(a)   (b)

Figure 3.6: Transverse slice of a reconstructed image of the dynamic FDK reconstruction result in (a) and the gold standard reconstruction of the phantom left ventricle at a relative heart phase of about 40 % and ROI (contour) used for evaluation in (b) (W 1900 HU, C 466 HU, slice thickness 1 mm). The ROI used for image quality metric measurements is shown as the red contour.

geometric reconstruction parameters as the motion-compensated reconstructions and the standard FDK reconstruction of the dynamic phantom, see Figure 3.6a. Let $f_{\mathrm{GS},\phi_k}(\boldsymbol{x})$ be the function, which returns the intensity value of the gold standard image for a certain heart phase, and $f_T(\boldsymbol{x}, \boldsymbol{s})$ the motion-compensated or standard FDK reconstructed image. The error as well as image quality metric were evaluated in a manually defined region of interest (ROI) around the ventricle. An example of the ROI is illustrated in Figure 3.6b.

- **Normalized Root Mean Square Error (nRMSE).** The nRMSE was used to quantify the 3-D reconstruction error of the motion-compensated reconstructions or standard FDK reconstructions compared to the gold standard FDK of the static phantom. The nRMSE can be computed as follows

$$\mathrm{nRMSE}_{\phi_k} \;=\; \zeta \cdot \sqrt{\frac{1}{|\Omega|} \sum_{x \in \Omega} \left(f_{\mathrm{GS},\phi_k}(\boldsymbol{x}) - f_T(\boldsymbol{x}, \boldsymbol{s}) \right)^2}, \;\; \text{with} \qquad (3.19)$$

$$\zeta \;=\; \frac{1}{\max_{x \in \Omega} \left(f_{\mathrm{GS},\phi_k}(\boldsymbol{x}) \right) - \min_{x \in \Omega} \left(f_{\mathrm{GS},\phi_k}(\boldsymbol{x}) \right)}, \qquad (3.20)$$

where $|\Omega|$ denotes the number of voxels inside the region of interest (ROI). All results were averaged over the heart phases, resulting in the overall nRMSE.

- **Universal Quality Index (UQI).** The 3-D image quality was evaluated with the universal image quality index (UQI) [Wang 02]. The UQI ranges from -1

to 1, where 1 is the best value achieved when $f_{\mathrm{GS},\phi_k}(\boldsymbol{x},\boldsymbol{s}) = f_T(\boldsymbol{x},\boldsymbol{s})$ for all $\boldsymbol{x}$. The UQI is defined as

$$\mathrm{UQI}_{\phi_k} = \frac{4 \cdot \sigma_{ff_{\mathrm{GS}}} \cdot \overline{f}_T \cdot \overline{f}_{\mathrm{GS},\phi_k}}{\left(\sigma_f^2 + \sigma_{f_{\mathrm{GS}}}^2\right)\left[(\overline{f}_T)^2 + (\overline{f}_{\mathrm{GS},\phi_k})^2\right]}, \tag{3.21}$$

where $\overline{f}_T$, $\overline{f}_{\mathrm{GS},\phi_k}$ represent the mean values, σ_f^2, $\sigma_{f_{\mathrm{GS}}}^2$ the variances, and $\sigma_{ff_{\mathrm{GS}}}$ the cross correlation inside the ROI Ω. For the overall UQI, all results were averaged over the heart phases ϕ_k.

Dice Similarity (DSC) Coefficient in 2-D Projection Space. In order to compare the reconstruction quality of the motion-compensated reconstruction algorithm, maximum intensity forward projections (MIPs) of the compensated LVs were generated. Binary mask images $\mathcal{B}_{\mathrm{FW}}(i,\phi_k)$ were created from the MIPs by thresholding, such that only the left ventricle is visible. A value equal to zero defines background and a non-zero value defines the ventricle shape. These binary images were compared to the segmented and binarized 2-D projections from which the original surface model and the MVF were built, denoted as $\mathcal{B}_{\mathrm{GS}}(i,\phi_k)$. The overlap of the binarized images and the segmented 2-D projections was analyzed with the Dice similarity coefficient (DSC) [Zou 04]. The DSC is defined in the range of $[0,1]$, where 0 means no overlap and 1 defines a perfect match between the two compared images. All results were averaged over the according projection images and the heart phases ϕ_k, resulting in the overall Dice coefficient. The DSC is defined as

$$\mathrm{DSC} = \frac{1}{K\,N} \sum_{k=1}^{K} \sum_{i=1}^{N} \sum_{i \in \phi_k} 2 \cdot \frac{|\mathcal{B}_{\mathrm{FW}}(i,\phi_k) \cdot \mathcal{B}_{\mathrm{GS}}(i,\phi_k)|}{|\mathcal{B}_{\mathrm{FW}}(i,\phi_k)| + |\mathcal{B}_{\mathrm{GS}}(i,\phi_k)|}, \tag{3.22}$$

with K denoting the number of heart phases and N the number of projection images.

Mean Contour Deviation ϵ in 2-D Projection Space. Since the motion-compensated reconstruction mainly improves the accuracy of the ventricle contour, the similarity of the contours was additionally evaluated. The binary contour images $\mathcal{C}_{\mathrm{FW}}(i,\phi_k)$ and $\mathcal{C}_{\mathrm{GS}}(i,\phi_k)$ of the binary masks of the forward projection $\mathcal{B}_{\mathrm{FW}}(i,\phi_k)$ and the gold standard projection $\mathcal{B}_{\mathrm{GS}}(i,\phi_k)$ were extracted. The contour $\mathcal{C}_{\mathrm{FW}}(i,\phi_k)$ is extracted by morphological operations from $\mathcal{B}_{\mathrm{FW}}(i,\phi_k)$. The contour $\mathcal{C}_{\mathrm{GS}}(i,\phi_k)$ is given by the 2-D bloodpool segmentation, see Section 3.3.2. In Figure 3.7a the boundary $\mathcal{C}_{\mathrm{GS}}(i,\phi_k)$ of the left ventricle is illustrated, which is used as gold standard. Figure 3.7b shows a binary contour image $\mathcal{C}_{\mathrm{FW}}(i,\phi_k)$.

A distance transform $\Phi(\mathcal{C}_{\mathrm{FW}}(i,\phi_k))$ of the binary contour images $\mathcal{C}_{\mathrm{FW}}(i,\phi_k)$ is defined by computing the Euclidean distance of every pixel to the contour $\mathcal{C}_{\mathrm{FW}}(i,\phi_k)$. An example of a distance transformed image $\Phi(\mathcal{C}_{\mathrm{FW}}(i,\phi_k))$ is shown in Figure 3.7c. An overlay of $\mathcal{C}_{\mathrm{GS}}(i,\phi_k)$ and $\Phi(\mathcal{C}_{\mathrm{FW}}(i,\phi_k))$ is shown in Figure 3.7d.

The distance transformed image is sampled only at the indices where $\mathcal{C}_{\mathrm{GS}}(i,\phi_k)$ is non-zero

$$\epsilon_{\mathcal{C}}(\phi_k) = \frac{1}{N_c} \sum_{i \in \phi_k} \sum_{n=1}^{N_c} \Phi(\mathcal{C}_{\mathrm{FW}}(i,\phi_k))_n, \tag{3.23}$$

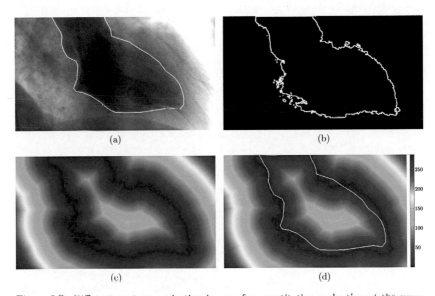

(a)   (b)

(c)   (d)

Figure 3.7: Different contour projection images for quantitative evaluation of the mean contour deviation in 2-D projection space. (a) Gold standard segmentation of the ventricle bloodpool in 2-D. (b) Extracted contour $\mathcal{C}_{\mathrm{FW}}(i, \phi_k)$ of the MIP projection image. (c) Euclidean distance transformed image $\Phi(\mathcal{C}_{\mathrm{FW}}(i, \phi_k))$. Dark color represents smaller distance and lighter color a larger contour distance. (d) Euclidean distance transformed image $\Phi(\mathcal{C}_{\mathrm{FW}}(i, \phi_k))$ overlaid with the contour $\mathcal{C}_{\mathrm{GS}}(i, \phi_k)$. For the computation of $\epsilon_{\mathcal{C}}(\phi_k)$ only the underlying values of $\Phi(\mathcal{C}_{\mathrm{FW}}(i, \phi_k))$ are used.

where N_c denotes the number of pixels where $\mathcal{C}_{GS}(i, \phi_k)$ is non-zero. All results were averaged over the heart phases, resulting in the overall mean contour deviation ϵ

$$\epsilon_{\mathcal{C}} = \sum_{k=1}^{K} \epsilon_{\mathcal{C}}(\phi_k), \qquad (3.24)$$

where a small $\epsilon_{\mathcal{C}}$ denotes similar contours over all heart phases.

3.5.1.3 Experimental Results

In this section, the quantitative results are presented for the five different datasets of the motion estimation and compensation approach.

Phantom Data. The quantitative 3-D results of the dynamic phantom model are presented in Table 3.2. The smallest nRMSE is obtained by the TPS and Shepard's method. The smoothed weighting function has a slightly larger error. The UQI for all motion-compensated reconstructions results in values around 99 %. In Table 3.3, the Dice and the contour deviation $\epsilon_{\mathcal{C}}$ in 2-D projection space for the phantom's left ventricle are reported. The TPS approach shows slightly superior, Shepard's method and the smoothed weighting function show equivalently good results. The contour deviation $\epsilon_{\mathcal{C}}$ of the TPS improved by about 1.91 pixels which corresponds to 1.18 mm compared to the standard FDK. The standard deviation is also much smaller with the TPS compared to the standard reconstruction. The Dice coefficient is not very sensitive and shows similar results between all interpolation methods as well as for the FDK reconstruction. In Figure 3.8, the results of the motion-compensated reconstructions of the phantom left ventricle using different interpolation methods are illustrated. There are minor visible differences in the endocardium border. All interpolation methods show deformation artifacts outside the region of interest, cf. Section 3.3.6.

Porcine Data. In Table 3.4, the results for the porcine left ventricle are reported. It can be seen that the best motion-compensated reconstruction can be achieved with the TPS interpolation method. The mean contour deviation $\epsilon_{\mathcal{C}}$ improved by about 0.97 pixels, which corresponds to 0.60 mm compared to the standard FDK reconstructions. The improvement is relatively small due to the fact that the pig had a poor ejection fraction of about 46 % and only small motion. In Figure 3.9, the results of different reconstructions, including the TPS reconstruction results of the porcine left ventricle are illustrated. The standard reconstruction in Figure 3.9a exhibits blurring around the LV. In Figure 3.9b, it can be observed that the ECG-gated reconstruction lacks LV structure and suffers from artifacts from the pigtail catheter. In comparison, the motion-compensated reconstruction shows an expansion in diastole and contraction in systole of the LV, see Figures 3.9c and 3.9d, respectively.

Clinical Data. In Table 3.5, the results for the human left ventricles are listed. The best motion-compensated reconstructions are clearly performed with the TPS for all three cases. The respective contour deviation $\epsilon_{\mathcal{C}}$ improved by about 8.45 pixels corresponding to 1.52 mm, about 4.32 pixels corresponding to 1.34 mm and about

Phantom p_0	nRMSE	UQI [%]
TPS	**0.047 ± 0.004**	98.5 ± 0.3
Shepard	**0.047 ± 0.004**	**98.9 ± 0.2**
Smoothed Weighting Fct.	0.048 ± 0.004	98.8 ± 0.2
Simple Averaging	0.050 ± 0.006	98.7 ± 0.2
Standard FDK	0.080 ± 0.019	96.2 ± 1.6

Table 3.2: The nRMSE and the UQI of the dynamic phantom model p_0. Expressed as mean value ± standard deviation. The best values are marked in bold.

Phantom p_0	Dice [pixel]	ϵ_C [pixel]	ϵ_C [mm]
TPS	**0.96 ± 0.02**	**2.75 ± 0.43**	**1.71 ± 0.27**
Shepard	0.95 ± 0.02	3.33 ± 0.31	2.06 ± 0.20
Smoothed Weighting Fct.	0.95 ± 0.02	3.33 ± 0.27	2.06 ± 0.17
Simple Averaging	0.94 ± 0.02	3.64 ± 0.33	2.26 ± 0.20
Standard FDK	0.94 ± 0.03	4.56 ± 1.91	2.89 ± 1.18

Table 3.3: Dice coefficient and mean contour deviation ϵ_C for the left ventricle of the phantom dataset p_0. Expressed as mean value ± standard deviation. The best values are marked in bold.

5.00 pixels corresponding to 1.55 mm compared to the standard FDK. The standard deviation is also much smaller with the TPS compared to the standard reconstructions. The widely used Shepard's method and the smoothed weighting function provides slightly inferior results compared to the TPS. The Dice coefficient shows similar results between all interpolation methods as well as for the FDK reconstruction, thus it is less sensitive compared to the contour deviation.

The standard reconstruction of case h_1 in Figure 3.10a exhibits blurring around the LV. In Figure 3.10b, it can be observed that the ECG-gated reconstruction lacks LV structure and suffers from artifacts. In comparison, the motion-compensated reconstruction using the TPS interpolation shows an expansion in diastole and contraction in systole of the LV, see Figures 3.10c and 3.10d, respectively. In Figure 3.11 the results of different interpolation schemes of the human left ventricle h_1 are illustrated. The motion-compensated reconstructions all show an expansion of the left ventricle, but slightly different shapes. The TPS reconstruction is closest to reality according to the quality measure ϵ_C.

Porcine p_{por}	Dice [pixel]	ϵ_C [pixel]	ϵ_C [mm]
TPS	**0.92 ± 0.01**	**3.67 ± 0.18**	**2.28 ± 0.11**
Shepard	**0.92 ± 0.01**	3.88 ± 0.19	2.39 ± 0.12
Smoothed Weighting Fct.	**0.92 ± 0.01**	4.50 ± 0.39	2.77 ± 0.24
Simple Averaging	**0.92 ± 0.01**	4.05 ± 0.20	2.51 ± 0.12
Standard FDK	0.90 ± 0.02	4.64 ± 0.49	2.88 ± 0.30

Table 3.4: Dice coefficient and mean contour deviation ϵ_C for the left ventricle of the porcine dataset p_{por}. Expressed as mean value ± standard deviation. The best values are marked in bold.

Human h_1	Dice [pixel]	ϵ_C [pixel]	ϵ_C [mm]
TPS	**0.93 ± 0.01**	**9.15 ± 1.22**	**1.65 ± 0.22**
Shepard	0.91 ± 0.02	10.29 ± 2.07	1.85 ± 0.33
Smoothed Weighting Fct.	0.91 ± 0.02	10.92 ± 3.02	1.97 ± 0.54
Simple Averaging	0.91 ± 0.03	11.74 ± 2.81	2.11 ± 0.51
Standard FDK	0.88 ± 0.03	17.60 ± 10.0	3.17 ± 1.80
Human h_2	**Dice [pixel]**	**ϵ[pixel]**	**ϵ [mm]**
TPS	**0.93 ± 0.01**	**6.70 ± 0.74**	**2.08 ± 0.23**
Shepard	**0.93 ± 0.02**	6.99 ± 1.37	2.17 ± 0.42
Smoothed Weighting Fct.	**0.93 ± 0.02**	7.17 ± 1.43	2.22 ± 0.44
Simple Averaging	**0.93 ± 0.02**	7.40 ± 1.98	2.29 ± 0.61
Standard FDK	0.89 ± 0.06	11.02 ± 5.80	3.42 ± 1.80
Human h_3	**Dice [pixel]**	**ϵ[pixel]**	**ϵ [mm]**
TPS	**0.88 ± 0.02**	**8.64 ± 0.98**	**2.68 ± 0.30**
Shepard	0.85 ± 0.03	12.13 ± 1.93	3.76 ± 0.60
Smoothed Weighting Fct.	0.85 ± 0.03	12.10 ± 1.88	3.75 ± 0.58
Simple Averaging	0.85 ± 0.03	12.38 ± 2.05	3.84 ± 1.19
Standard FDK	0.83 ± 0.06	13.64 ± 5.81	4.23 ± 1.80

Table 3.5: Dice coefficient and mean contour deviation ϵ_C for the left ventricle of the human datasets h_1–h_3. Expressed as mean value ± standard deviation. The best values are marked in bold.

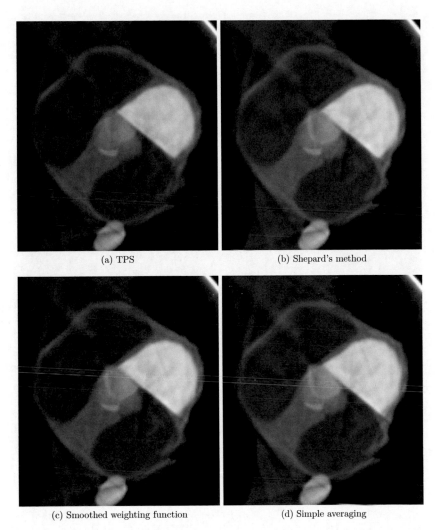

(a) TPS   (b) Shepard's method

(c) Smoothed weighting function   (d) Simple averaging

Figure 3.8: Detail of an axial slice of the motion-compensated reconstruction images of the phantom left ventricle p_0 at a heart phase of about 40 % using different interpolation methods (W 1900 HU, C 466 HU, slice thickness 1 mm).

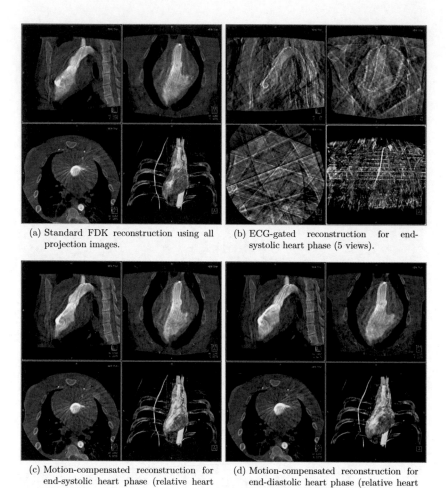

(a) Standard FDK reconstruction using all projection images.

(b) ECG-gated reconstruction for end-systolic heart phase (5 views).

(c) Motion-compensated reconstruction for end-systolic heart phase (relative heart phase of about 30 %).

(d) Motion-compensated reconstruction for end-diastolic heart phase (relative heart phase of about 95 %).

Figure 3.9: Every image shows multi-planar reconstruction images (long axis view top left and right, short axis view bottom left) and volume rendering (bottom right) of the reconstruction results of the porcine left ventricle (W 1260 HU, C 1075 HU, slice thickness 0.85 mm). The ECG-gated reconstruction was windowed to be visually comparable. The image data was provided by Assoc. Prof. Rebecca Fahrig, Ph.D., RSL, Department of Radiology, Stanford University.

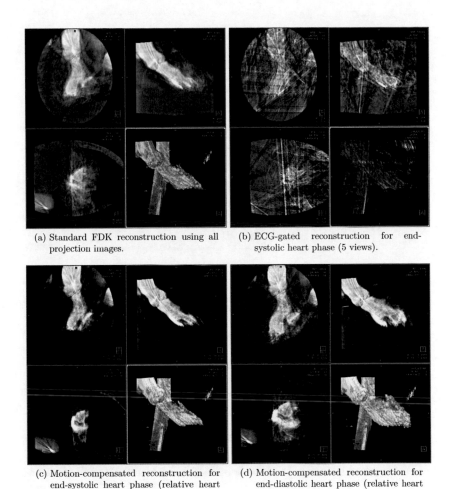

(a) Standard FDK reconstruction using all projection images.

(b) ECG-gated reconstruction for end-systolic heart phase (5 views).

(c) Motion-compensated reconstruction for end-systolic heart phase (relative heart phase of about 20 %).

(d) Motion-compensated reconstruction for end-diastolic heart phase (relative heart phase of about 70 %).

Figure 3.10: Every image shows multi-planar reconstruction images (long axis view top left and right, short axis view bottom left) and volume rendering (bottom right) of the reconstruction results of the human left ventricle h_1 with the TPS interpolation (W 3000 HU, C 1200 HU, slice thickness 3.0 mm). The ECG-gated reconstruction was windowed to be visually comparable. The image data was provided by Dr. med. Schultz from the Thoraxcenter, Erasmus MC Rotterdam, The Netherlands.

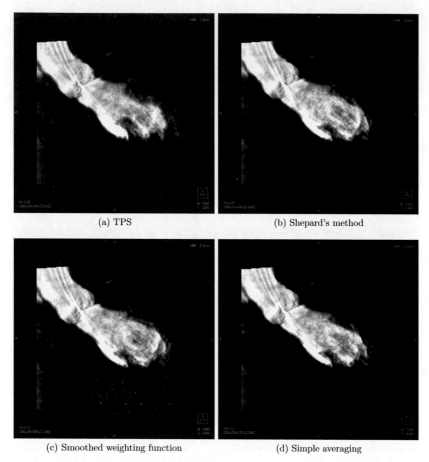

(a) TPS   (b) Shepard's method

(c) Smoothed weighting function   (d) Simple averaging

Figure 3.11: Coronal slice of the reconstruction images (long axis view) of the motion-compensated reconstruction results of the human left ventricle h_1 and an end-diastolic heart phase of about 70 % (W 3000 HU, C 1200 HU, slice thickness 3.0 mm). The image data was provided by Dr. med. Schultz from the Thoraxcenter, Erasmus MC Rotterdam, The Netherlands.

3.5.2   Wall Motion Analysis

In this section, the wall motion parameters presented in Section 3.4 are computed and analyzed on specifically designed phantom and clinical patient data. Furthermore, the individual steps of the surface model generation and the influence on the wall motion parameters is evaluated in more detail on the phantom datasets. The analysis is done with respect to the sensitivity of the size variation of the left ventricle and the perspective change of the rotating C-arm system.

3.5.2.1   Datasets

In order to evaluate if the parameters presented in Section 3.4 are clinical significant, different phantoms were created with different pathological defects. The analysis framework was tested on eight clinical datasets without any clinical indication. Two of the clinical datasets (h_2 and h_3) were already used for the evaluation of the motion estimation and compensation approach in Section 3.5.1.

Ventricular Phantoms.   The analysis presented here has been applied to specifically designed LV surface models generated from a cardiac phantom [Maie 12, Mlle 13b, Maie 13], which is similarly designed to the widely used 4-D XCAT phantom [Sega 08]. The phantom is defined by cubic B-splines and can be tessellated to generate a triangulated mesh for every time point. The splines can be sampled at any number of points. In our experiments, we sampled the spline at about about 870 surface points. The simulated acquisition protocol uses a total of 133 projection images with a size of 1240 × 960 pixels and a pixel resolution of 0.3 mm. The dynamic LV surface models were simulated over 5 s at a heart rate of 60 bpm. Five different surface phantoms were generated with various contraction dynamics and considered as ground truth (GT), denoted as $p_{1,\mathrm{GT}}$–$p_{5,\mathrm{GT}}$. For the evaluation of the phantom data, dynamic phantom meshes were generated as described in Sections 3.3.1 to 3.3.4. The meshes had $\Gamma_c = 545$ control points uniformly distributed over the left ventricle and are denoted as p_1–p_5. The 2-D segmentation of the phantom data cannot be used to validate the bloodpool segmentation since the segmentation of clinical LV acquisitions and the segmentation of phantom simulations are not comparable. Therefore, the GT 2-D segmentation of the left ventricles were used to generate the dynamic LV meshes.

Modeling of Pathological Motion Patterns.   As mentioned previously, a cubic B-spline is used to model the 3-D anatomy as well as the motion path [Maie 12]. The simulation of left ventricular phantom datasets is already described in Müller et al. [Mlle 13b]. For every normalized time point $t \in [0, 1]$ of the whole scan, there exists a 2-D spline surface $s(t) \in [0, 1]^2$. The normalized time points t during the scan are defined by the mapping from the projection index i to

$$t = \frac{i - 1}{N - 1}, \tag{3.25}$$

where N denotes the number of projection images. Each spline is defined by control points $c \in \mathbb{R}^2$ with a one-to-one mapping from 3-D coordinates $C \in \mathbb{R}^3$ to the 2-D control points c given by the 4-D XCAT phantom [Sega 99, Sega 08]. In order to incorporate a motion defect, a region in which the motion is pathological has to be defined. Here, a box $\mathcal{B}$ is defined located at the lateral wall, within the coordinate system of the heart, i.e. a local coordinate system where the z-axis is aligned with the principal axis of the heart. Each spline control point C is clipped against the volume $\mathcal{B}$, generating a list $\mathcal{C}_{path}$ of control points inside the pathological volume, where the complete set of all control points is denoted as $\mathcal{C}$. During the tessellation procedure $T(s) : \mathbb{R}^2 \to \mathbb{R}^3$, the 2-D spline surface points s are assigned to a 3-D coordinate $x(t) = T(s)$. This is done for each normalized time point t of the whole scan. In order to allow for a smoother transition between $\mathcal{B}$ and the healthy LV surface, a flexibility parameter σ is introduced. A larger value of σ results in a smooth defect, while a small value yields sharp transitions between pathological and normal tissue. The model incorporates two kinds of motion defects: akinetic and dyskinetic wall motion. The akinetic motion defect prevents contraction or inward motion of the heart in the affected area. A delayed motion is a contradictory movement of the heart. The motion defects can be controlled by a phase shift parameter $\delta \in [0, 1]$. The deformed 3-D coordinate can then be computed as

$$x_{path}(t) = (1 - w_G(s(t))) \cdot T(s(t)) + w_G(s(t)) \cdot T(s(t - \delta)), \qquad (3.26)$$

$$w_G(s) = \frac{\sum_{c \in \mathcal{C}_{path}} w'_G(s, c)}{\sum_{c \in \mathcal{C}} w'_G(s, c)}, \qquad (3.27)$$

$$w'_G(s, c) = e^{-\frac{1}{2\sigma^2}\|s - c\|_2^2}. \qquad (3.28)$$

The Gaussian basis function $w'_G(s, c)$ gives a small weight to control points far away from the current spline surface point s and a higher weight to close control points. Effectively, $x_{path}(t)$ is a linear combination between the transformed spline point s at the current time t and at a time point $t - \delta$. An akinetic motion defect can be realized by setting $\delta = t - t_0$. In our experiments, we set $t_0 = 0$. Hence, the magnitude of the motion in the pathological volume is minimal compared to the motion of the remaining LV. A dyskinetic defect models a shift in the motion phase. This is achieved by setting δ to a fixed value, given as percentage of the heart cycle. Consequently, $x_{path}(t)$ is generated from the transformed spline points at the current time and at an earlier time with a fixed phase shift. As a result, the motion in the pathological volume is delayed compared to the motion of the remaining LV.

Five different phantom datasets were simulated. The LV surface model p_1 exhibits normal dynamics, three LVs suffered from a temporal contraction shift on the lateral wall of 10 % (p_2, $\delta = 0.1$, $\sigma = 0.1$), 20 % (p_3, $\delta = 0.2$, $\sigma = 0.1$) and 30 % (p_4, $\delta = 0.3$, $\sigma = 0.1$) relative to the heart cycle. Another LV (p_5, $\sigma = 0.05$) had an induced wall defect on the lateral LV wall, i.e. no movement at the lateral wall. All LV surface meshes and defined parameters are publicly available for download[3]. In Figure 3.12, the phantom meshes for $p_{1,GT}$, $p_{5,GT}$ and p_1 are illustrated for both end-diastolic and end-systolic phases.

The 3-D volumes of the different GT phantoms are plotted in Figure 3.13. The different contraction shifts as well as the wall motion defect are clearly visible in the curves. A more detailed analysis of the volume curves of the affected segments is

---

[3]http://conrad.stanford.edu/data/heart

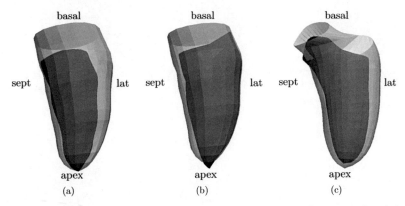

Figure 3.12: Wall motion of the LV surface models at end-diastole (transparent) and the solid surface representing the surface mesh at end-systole. (a) Anterior view of the phantom surfaces $p_{1,GT}$ with normal contraction behavior and in (b) of the phantom surface $p_{5,GT}$ with the lateral wall defect. (c) Anterior view of the estimated surfaces p_1.

given in Table 3.6. For the affected segments (segments 5, 6, 11, 12 and 16) the mean phase of maximal contraction $\phi_{s,\max}$ is computed. The phase shift for every phantom is given as $\widetilde{\delta}$ and the relation to the parameter δ is denoted as ϵ_δ. The motion of the surface points is influenced by the Gaussian function and the flexibility parameter σ, thus, the phase shift or akinesis is not constant over the pathological region. Hence, the maximal phase shift ($\max \widetilde{\delta}$) and its relation to the parameter δ is also given in Table 3.6.

In Table 3.7, the motion parameters for the different GT phantom datasets are given ($p_{1,GT}$–$p_{5,GT}$). It can be seen that the normal phantom has an SDI of 4.16 % which is in the upper normal range. In Figure 3.14a, the Hammer map of $\phi_{c,\max}$ of

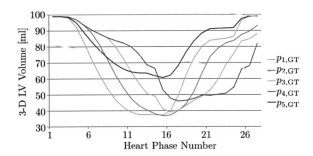

Figure 3.13: 3-D LV volume curves of the different phantoms ($p_{1,GT}$–$p_{5,GT}$).

Dataset	$\phi_{s,\mathrm{max}}$ for affected segments	$\tilde{\delta}$	ϵ_δ to param. δ	max $\tilde{\delta}$	ϵ_δ to param. δ
$p_{1,\mathrm{GT}}$	0.52 ± 0.00	-	-	-	-
$p_{2,\mathrm{GT}}$	0.60 ± 0.02	0.08	0.02	0.11	0.01
$p_{3,\mathrm{GT}}$	0.67 ± 0.03	0.15	0.05	0.18	0.02
$p_{4,\mathrm{GT}}$	0.79 ± 0.02	0.27	0.03	0.29	0.01
$p_{5,\mathrm{GT}}$	n.a.	n.a.	n.a.	n.a.	n.a.

Table 3.6: Contraction times of affected segments $\phi_{s,\mathrm{max}}$, resulting phase shifts ($\tilde{\delta}$), the relation of $\tilde{\delta}$ to the parameter δ denoted as ϵ_δ are given. The maximal phase shift (max $\tilde{\delta}$) is also given for the phantom GT datasets.

Dataset	phase shift	HR [bpm]	EF [%]	SDI [%]
$p_{1,\mathrm{GT}}$	0 % [lateral]	60	62.37	4.16
$p_{2,\mathrm{GT}}$	10 % [lateral]	60	62.97	5.22
$p_{3,\mathrm{GT}}$	20 % [lateral]	60	60.40	6.47
$p_{4,\mathrm{GT}}$	30 % [lateral]	60	53.65	12.74
$p_{5,\mathrm{GT}}$	0 % [defect lateral]	60	38.70	5.05

Table 3.7: Heart rate (HR), ejection fraction (EF), and the systolic dyssynchrony index (SDI) of the GT phantom datasets.

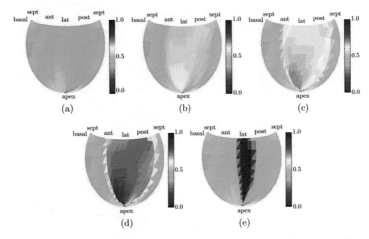

Figure 3.14: Ground truth Hammer map of $\phi_{c,\max}$ of the phantom dataset with (a) normal, synchronous LV contraction $(p_{1,\mathrm{GT}})$, (b) relative phase shift of 10 % on lateral wall $(p_{2,\mathrm{GT}})$, (c) relative phase shift of 20 % on lateral wall $(p_{3,\mathrm{GT}})$, (d) relative phase shift of 30 % on lateral wall $(p_{4,\mathrm{GT}})$ and (e) lateral wall defect $(p_{5,\mathrm{GT}})$.

$p_{1,\mathrm{GT}}$ is illustrated. It can be seen that the phase to maximal contraction is uniformly distributed over the LV. The 3DFS$_c$ Hammer map is given in Figure 3.15a. On the lateral wall of $p_{1,\mathrm{GT}}$, the 3DFS$_i$ is about 0.4. In comparison, $p_{3,\mathrm{GT}}$ and $p_{4,\mathrm{GT}}$ with the induced lateral phase shift are classified to have a mild or even severe dysfunction with an SDI ≥ 6.0 % [Sach 11]. The phantom $p_{2,\mathrm{GT}}$ has a small phase shift and, hence, only a slightly increased SDI value. In Figures 3.14b through 3.14d, the Hammer maps of $\phi_{c,\max}$ of $(p_{2,\mathrm{GT}} - p_{4,\mathrm{GT}})$ are illustrated. The increase in the phase to maximal contraction is visible on the lateral wall. The 3DFS$_c$ decreases compared to $p_{1,\mathrm{GT}}$, cf. Figures 3.15b through 3.15d. It can be seen that the phase shifts affect the whole ventricle since the time point of the end-diastole and end-systole differs compared to $p_{1,\mathrm{GT}}$. From Figure 3.13, it can be observed that the systolic phase is shifted towards the end of one cardiac cycle, therefore, the "normal/healthy" wall part is measured too early and the "impaired" wall motion is measured too late. For phantom $p_{5,\mathrm{GT}}$, the defect on the lateral wall is visible in the Hammer maps at the lateral wall, cf. Figure 3.14e and Figure 3.15e. The 3DFS$_c$ drops to about 0.0 at the lateral wall for the wall defect. The small EF of about 39 % is additionally an indicator for a wall dysfunction. The SDI shows no abnormal behavior due to its dependence on averaged volumetric information inside the individual segments. The affected segments still contract slightly and show a contraction $\phi_{s,\max}$. However, the Hammer map of $\phi_{c,\max}$ identifies the wall motion defect.

Clinical Data.   Patient datasets were acquired on an Artis zee and Artis zeego C-arm system (Siemens AG, Healthcare Sector, Forchheim, Germany) at two clinical sites (Universitätsklinikum Erlangen, Germany and at the Thoraxcenter, Erasmus

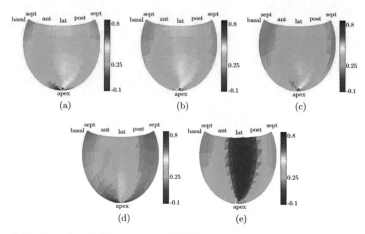

Figure 3.15: Ground truth Hammer map of $3DFS_c$ of the phantom dataset with (a) normal, synchronous LV contraction ($p_{1,GT}$), (b) relative phase shift of 10 % on lateral wall ($p_{2,GT}$), (c) relative phase shift of 20 % on lateral wall ($p_{3,GT}$), (d) relative phase shift of 30 % on lateral wall ($p_{4,GT}$) and (e) lateral wall defect ($p_{5,GT}$).

MC Rotterdam, the Netherlands). The acquisition protocol is based on the description in Section 3.2. Two different protocols were used: the first protocol with a number of 133 projection images at a frame rate of 30 fps with a size of 960 × 960 pixels and a pixel resolution of 0.31 mm over 200° and an angular increment of 1.5°/f. The source-to-detector distance was 120 cm and the source-to-isocenter was 78 cm, resulting in a resolution of 0.2 mm in the isocenter. The contrast agent was administered with 15 ml/s over 5 s scan time and 1 s X-ray delay. The second protocol with a number of 248 projection images with a frame rate of 60 fps with a size of 480 × 480 pixels with a pixel resolution of 0.6 mm over 200° and an angular increment of 0.8°/f. The source-to-detector distance was 120 cm and the source-to-isocenter was 78 cm, resulting in a resolution of 0.4 mm in the isocenter. Here, the contrast agent was also administered directly into the left ventricle at 10 ml/s over 5 s scan time also with an X-ray delay of 1 s. The generated surface models consisted of a different number of heart phases $K = 26.5 \pm 6.70$ dependent on the frames per cardiac cycle and hence the patient's heart rate. In general, the number of heart phases needs to be smaller than the number of images per heart cycle. In the experiments, not less than 5 projection images were used for the reconstruction of each heart phase. The surface meshes consist of 609 points equally distributed over the left ventricle and the outflow tract, and $P_c = 545$ control points define the left ventricle. The examining cardiologists diagnosed no pathological LV dynamics on all eight patient datasets.

Dataset	ϵ_p [mm]
p_1	1.11 ± 0.18
p_2	2.12 ± 1.18
p_3	1.25 ± 0.30
p_4	1.31 ± 0.29
p_5	1.21 ± 0.25
Mean	1.40 ± 0.41

Table 3.8: Mean point-to-mesh error ϵ_p with ± standard deviation for the five different phantom datasets averaged over all mesh points and all time steps .

3.5.2.2 Experimental Results

In this section, the results for the generated phantom datasets and the clinical datasets are presented.

Phantom Data.   For the phantom data, the accuracy of the individual steps to generate the surface meshes are evaluated. Furthermore, the computed wall motion parameters are compared to the ground truth parameters.

Mesh Error Analysis.   In Table 3.8, an average point-to-mesh error ϵ_p is used for measuring the difference between the estimated meshes (p_1–p_5) and the ground truth meshes ($p_{1,\text{GT}}$–$p_{5,\text{GT}}$) over all time points. A final point-to-mesh error of 1.40 ± 0.41 mm over all phantom datasets is achieved. It can be seen that the phase shift of 10 % of p_2 results in the highest deviation. A reason for this may be that the small deviation in the lateral wall is not visible in a large number of 2-D projection images which are used to built the dynamic model. Overall, when setting the point-to-mesh error in relation to the ventricle size, defined as twice the distance to the long axis, the percentage error is about 3 %. A small mismatch between the estimated meshes p_1–p_5 and the ground truth $p_{1,\text{GT}}$–$p_{5,\text{GT}}$ is due to the smoother appearance and the different mesh topology of the generated meshes, cf. Figure 3.12.

Heart Phase Identification Analysis.   In order to evaluate the accuracy of the heart phase identification using the 2-D bloodpool segmentation, the five phantom datasets are used. In Table 3.9, the error between the ground truth heart phase of p_1–p_5 and the estimated heart phases is given. For the phantom experiments a number of $K = 27$ bins was chosen. The mean error is denoted with ϵ_ϕ given in relative heart phases between $[0, 1]$. The overall mean error ϵ_ϕ of all phantom datasets is 0.06 ± 0.02. Furthermore, the mean error ϵ_{ϕ_k} of the binned heart phase is also given. The overall mean ϵ_{ϕ_k} is less than one heart phase bin and results in 0.78 ± 0.28. A scatter plot of the ground truth heart phase number and the estimated heart phase is illustrated in Figure 3.16a. A small number of outliers can be seen of maximum 2 bins at diastolic heart phases. The small mismatch may be due to the longer lasting

Dataset	K	ϵ_ϕ	ϵ_{ϕ_k}	ϱ_π	ϱ_{π_n}
p_1	27	0.06 ± 0.16	0.60 ± 0.59	0.82	0.99
p_2	27	0.05 ± 0.14	0.51 ± 0.60	0.80	0.99
p_3	27	0.04 ± 0.14	0.74 ± 0.79	0.74	0.98
p_4	27	0.07 ± 0.16	1.24 ± 1.26	0.67	0.94
p_5	27	0.08 ± 0.18	0.80 ± 0.78	0.69	0.99
Mean	27	0.06 ± 0.02	0.78 ± 0.28	0.74 ± 0.07	0.98 ± 0.02

Table 3.9: Accuracy and correlation of the heart phase identification for the phantom datasets. The mean relative heart phase error ϵ_ϕ and the mean error of the binned heart phase ϵ_{ϕ_k} are shown. The correlation coefficients between the original segmented 2-D bloodpool signal $\pi(i)$ and the 3-D volume $\Pi(i)$ are given as ϱ_π. The correlation coefficients between the normalized 2-D bloodpool signal $\pi_n(i)$ and $\Pi(i)$ are given as ϱ_{π_n}.

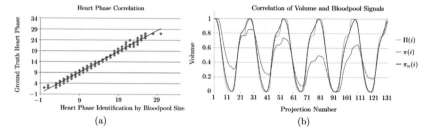

(a)   (b)

Figure 3.16: (a) Correlation between heart phases identified by 2-D bloodpool size and the ground truth heart phase of phantom p_1. (b) 3-D volume signal $\Pi(i)$, the 2-D segmented bloodpool signal $\pi(i)$ and the normalized bloodpool signal $\pi_n(i)$ of phantom dataset p_1.

diastole where the 3-D volume is almost constant and hence the detection of the ED phase can vary slightly.

In order to evaluate if the bloodpool size variation due to cardiac phase variation can be distinguished from perspective size variations due to the rotation of the C-arm, a correlation coefficient ϱ_π between the original segmented 2-D bloodpool signal $\pi(i)$ and the 3-D volume signal $\Pi(i)$ is computed. The mean correlation ϱ_π for all five phantom datasets is 0.74 ± 0.07. However, in order to identify the respective heart phase, the bloodpool signal is normalized as described in Section 3.3.3. Therefore, the correlation coefficient ϱ_{π_n} is also given for the normalized bloodpool signal $\pi_n(i)$ and the 3-D volume signal $\Pi(i)$. Here, the mean correlation coefficient results in 0.98 ± 0.02 for p_1–p_5. Thus, the change in the bloodpool size due to the cardiac phase can be distinguished from the perspective size variations due to the normalization step. The bloodpool signal $\pi(i)$, the normalized bloodpool $\pi_n(i)$ and the 3-D volume signal $\Pi(i)$ of phantom p_1 are illustrated in Figure 3.16b.

Dataset	$\phi_{s,\max}$ for affected segments	$\phi_{s,\max}$ error to GT	max $\tilde{\delta}$ error to GT
p_1	0.45 ± 0.03	0.07	0.02
p_2	0.48 ± 0.03	0.12	0.13
p_3	0.58 ± 0.03	0.09	0.08
p_4	0.70 ± 0.05	0.09	0.04
p_5	n.a.	n.a.	n.a.
Mean		0.09 ± 0.02	0.07 ± 0.05

Table 3.10: Contraction times of affected segments $\phi_{s,\max}$, the error compared to the GT $\phi_{s,\max}$ given in Table 3.6 and the error between the maximal phase shifts (max $\tilde{\delta}$).

Motion Analysis.   In Table 3.10, the quantitative results for the estimated phase shifts of (p_1-p_5) are given. The deviation between (p_1-p_5) and $(p_{1,\mathrm{GT}}-p_{5,\mathrm{GT}})$ is stated in column three. The overall deviation of the mean phase shift is about 9 % of a cardiac cycle and for the maximal phase shift about 7 % of a cardiac cycle.

The results for the motion analysis parameter for the phantom meshes compared to the GT meshes are given in Table 3.11. In general it can be seen that the estimated meshes underestimate the EF and the SDI values in most datasets. However, the tendency between the estimated and the ground truth values are similar and show the same noticeable pathologies as the GT values. In Figure 3.17, the Hammer maps with $\phi_{c,\max}$ for p_1-p_5 are shown. For dataset p_1, the Hammer map (Figure 3.17a) shows a homogeneous distribution as in the GT map of $p_{1,\mathrm{GT}}$ in Figure 3.14a. For p_2-p_4, the increase of the motion deficit is visible on the lateral wall. For p_2 and p_3 a smaller band on the lateral wall is delayed compared to the GT LV meshes. The phantom p_3 with 30 % phase shift in Figure 3.17d shows a high correlation with the GT Hammer map in Figure 3.14d. For the phantom with the lateral wall defect, a reduction of the motionless band can be identified. A small overshoot is visible close to the lateral wall, see Figure 3.14e and Figure 3.17e. The small deviation of the GT meshes and the estimated meshes are given in the difference $\phi_{c,\max}$ Hammer maps in Figure 3.18. For p_5 the slight overshoots at the lateral wall are visible. The 3DFS$_c$ Hammer maps are illustrated in Figure 3.19. In Figure 3.20, the corresponding difference maps are given. They show that the highest deviation between the meshes occurs around the apex region.

Clinical Data   The clinical data was evaluated with respect to motion analysis parameter.

Motion Analysis.   The results for the eight patient datasets are given in Table 3.12 (h_2-h_9). It can be observed that all patients are classified as healthy using the SDI according to [Kape 05, Sach 11]. An example of the surface meshes of dataset h_8 is shown in Figure 3.21a and the dynamic contraction curves for each segment's subvolume for dataset h_8 are shown in Figure 3.21b. All segments contract synchronously,

Dataset	EF [%]	σ to GT	SDI [%]	σ to GT
p_1	62.39	0.02	3.68	-0.61
p_2	59.63	-3.34	3.50	-1.72
p_3	54.11	-6.29	5.08	-1.39
p_4	49.16	-4.49	9.42	-3.32
p_5	41.49	2.79	6.16	1.11
Mean		3.39 ± 2.31		1.60 ± 1.03

Table 3.11: Ejection fraction (EF) and systolic dyssynchrony index (SDI) of the phantom datasets and the deviation σ to the ground truth phantom datasets.

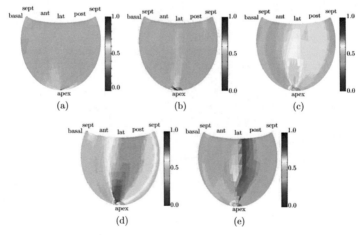

Figure 3.17: Estimated Hammer map of $\phi_{c,\text{max}}$ of the phantom dataset with (a) normal, synchronous LV contraction (p_1), (b) relative phase shift of 10 % on lateral wall (p_2), (c) relative phase shift of 20 % on lateral wall (p_3), (d) relative phase shift of 30 % on lateral wall (p_4) and (e) lateral wall defect (p_5).

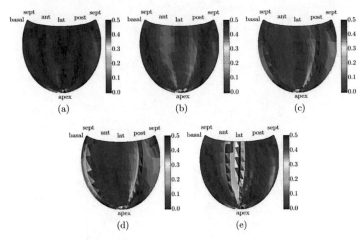

Figure 3.18: Difference Hammer map of $\phi_{c,\max}$ of the ground truth and the estimated phantom dataset with (a) normal, synchronous LV contraction ($|p_1\text{-}p_{1,\mathrm{GT}}|$), (b) relative phase shift of 10 % on lateral wall ($|p_2\text{-}p_{2,\mathrm{GT}}|$), (c) relative phase shift of 20 % on lateral wall ($|p_3\text{-}p_{3,\mathrm{GT}}|$), (d) relative phase shift of 30 % on lateral wall ($|p_4\text{-}p_{4,\mathrm{GT}}|$) and (e) lateral wall defect ($|p_5\text{-}p_{5,\mathrm{GT}}|$).

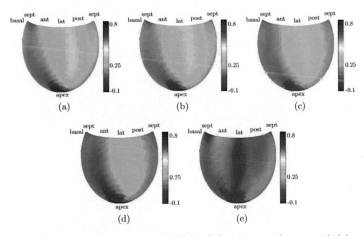

Figure 3.19: Estimated Hammer map of $3\mathrm{DFS}_c$ of the phantom dataset with (a) normal, synchronous LV contraction (p_1), (b) relative phase shift of 10 % on lateral wall (p_2), (c) relative phase shift of 20 % on lateral wall (p_3), (d) relative phase shift of 30 % on lateral wall (p_4) and (e) lateral wall defect (p_5).

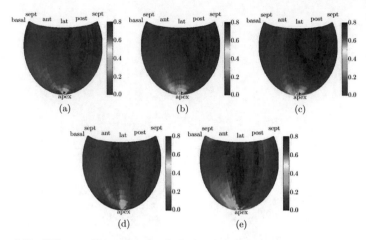

Figure 3.20: Difference Hammer map of 3DFS$_c$ of the ground truth and the estimated phantom dataset with (a) normal, synchronous LV contraction ($|p_1\text{-}p_{1,\mathrm{GT}}|$), (b) relative phase shift of $10\,\%$ on lateral wall ($|p_2\text{-}p_{2,\mathrm{GT}}|$), (c) relative phase shift of $20\,\%$ on lateral wall ($|p_3\text{-}p_{3,\mathrm{GT}}|$), (d) relative phase shift of $30\,\%$ on lateral wall ($|p_4\text{-}p_{4,\mathrm{GT}}|$) and (e) lateral wall defect ($|p_5\text{-}p_{5,\mathrm{GT}}|$).

hence, the curves have almost the same $\phi_{s,\mathrm{max}}$ and a small SDI. In Figure 3.22a, $\phi_{c,\mathrm{max}}$ of dataset h_8 is shown. The maximal contraction phase is homogeneously distributed over the whole LV. Small hypokinetic regions are indicated by mesh points close to the apex point, as visible in the 3DFS$_c$ Hammer map of dataset h_8 in Figure 3.22b, as well as on the 3-D overlay in Figure 3.22c. The motion close to the apex is small compared to the remaining mesh, hence this area is sensitive to errors introduced by the 2-D segmentation, position of the points to the principal axis $\boldsymbol{n}_1$ and the consistency of data from different heart cycles.

Principle Axis Alignment.   The PCA does not necessarily yield an axis $\boldsymbol{n}_1$ which passes through the apex, as the LV is not necessarily symmetric. For that reason the local coordinate system is rotated in order to align $\boldsymbol{n}_1$ with the long axis given by the mid point of the mitral valve and the apex. These points are detected by the initial model-based surface mesh fitting on the non-gated C-arm CT volume [Zhen 08]. During deformation of the initial mesh to fit the 2-D angiographic data, the topology of the 3-D mesh is preserved, and the apex and mitral valve points (mitral valve annulus) are consistent over the whole cardiac cycle. The rotation of the axis $\boldsymbol{n}_1$ to the long axis with the rotation angle $\angle_{\mathrm{rot}}$ can be performed accurately. In Table 3.13, the rotation angles for the clinical datasets are given.

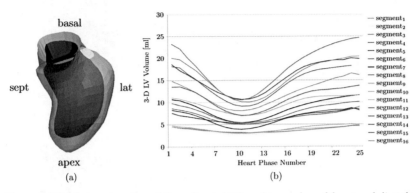

(a)   (b)

Figure 3.21: (a) Anterior view of the estimated LV surface meshes of h_8 at end-diastole (transparent) and the solid surface representing the surface mesh at end-systole. (b) 3-D LV volume curves for each segment of dataset h_8 over the different heart phases.

	Heart rate [bpm]	EF [%]	SV [ml]	EDV [ml]	ESV [ml]	SDI [%]
Human h_2	62.9 ± 2.9	58.73	65.14	110.91	45.77	2.88
Human h_3	55.3 ± 9.3	62.33	89.07	142.91	53.84	3.42
Human h_4	59.9 ± 0.4	72.26	80.49	111.39	30.90	2.08
Human h_5	58.3 ± 0.3	50.98	91.57	179.62	88.06	2.85
Human h_6	88.6 ± 25.0	70.58	30.12	42.68	12.56	2.48
Human h_7	73.4 ± 8.4	63.08	82.36	130.55	48.20	1.22
Human h_8	63.9 ± 0.8	50.32	96.42	191.61	95.20	1.79
Human h_9	52.7 ± 0.5	56.69	95.89	169.13	73.24	1.79

Table 3.12: Physiological data parameters extracted from the surface models: ejection fraction (EF), stroke volume (SV), end-diastolic volume (EDV), end-systolic volume (ESV), systolic dyssynchrony index (SDI) of the clinical patient datasets.

Dataset	h_2	h_3	h_4	h_5	h_6	h_7	h_8	h_9	$\overline{\angle}_{rot}$
$\angle_{rot}$ [°]	9.14	7.46	6.33	8.37	14.86	17.92	16.54	16.36	12.12 ± 4.73

Table 3.13: Rotation angle variation of the clinical datasets.

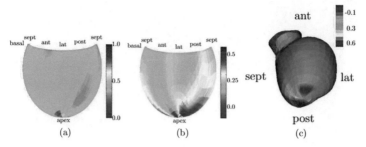

Figure 3.22: Hammer map of (a) $\phi_{c,\text{max}}$ of dataset h_8, (b) 3DFS$_c$ of dataset h_8 with visible abnormalities of the LV surface around the apex region. (c) Color overlay of the 3DFS$_c$ onto the endocardial LV surface of dataset h_8.

3.6   Challenges

Both, the motion interpolation result and the motion-compensated reconstruction as well as the wall motion analysis is dependent on the robustness and stability of the extracted surface model. The surface model extraction method is robust with respect to higher heart rates up to 100 bpm or even more. The porcine model had a heart rate of about 100 bpm. However, if the heart beat is quite arrhythmic, the assignment of the projection images to a certain heart phase becomes ambiguous and thus the generation of the dynamic surface model is not unique. This problem was minored by using the 2-D bloodpool as identification of the relative heart phase instead of the ECG-signal. However, it is still a challenging task, since the 2-D bloodpool can be similar but the motion state of the heart can be different.

For the wall motion analysis, spatial resolution is limited by the number of projection images used for the dynamic mesh fitting process. Here, the scan time for the clinical patient datasets was 5 s, resulting in 5 projections per heart phase with a heart rate of 60 bpm. By increasing the scan time to 8 s, a total of 8 projection images might be used to regularize the dynamic LV mesh generation and hence to increase the spatial resolution, but a longer scan time implies a higher radiation dose and a higher contrast burden for the patient.

As previously mentioned, the motion close to the apex is small compared to the remaining mesh, hence this area is sensitive to errors introduced by the 2-D segmentation. In general, the original LV surface is quite structured due to the papillary muscles. However, a smooth boundary is extracted from the 2-D projections for the surface mesh generation, thus, 2-D segmentation errors occur. It is known that during the surface generation, the assumption of motion along the surface-normal is reasonable for the middle and basal LV segments, but not good for the LV apex, since many intersections in the trajectories of mesh points around the apex can occur. In a first clinical prototype, the motion in the apex could be grayed out for the visualization in order to avoid misleading the cardiologist. In the future, the issue can be mitigated by using a learned prior mean motion trajectory from dynamic cardiac CT sequences [Chen 13c]. Up to now, the evaluation of the presented wall motion analysis framework is a feasibility study. The next step in the evaluation of the framework is a validation of the extracted parameters compared to parameters estimated from MRI or 3-D echocardiography.

3.7   Summary and Conclusions

In this chapter, a whole framework for left ventricular tomographic reconstruction and wall motion analysis was presented. Dynamic surface models were generated from the 2-D X-ray images acquired during a short scan of a C-arm scanner using the 2-D bloodpool information. The acquisition time was 5 s and the patient had a normal sinus rhythm. Due to the slow rotation speed of the C-arm, no valuable retrospective ECG-gated reconstructions were possible. The dynamic surface LV model comprises a sparse motion vector field on the surface, but in order to perform a tomographic motion-compensated reconstruction, a dense motion vector field is required. Therefore, the influence of different motion interpolation methods was investigated, a thin-plate spline, Shepard's method, a smoothed weighting based approach and simple averaging were used. The best quantitative results (Dice coefficient, mean contour deviation) for a phantom, a porcine and three human datasets were achieved using the TPS interpolation approach. Shepard's method and the smoothed weighting function might be a good compromise between computational efficiency and accuracy. The framework also enables the analysis of the contraction behavior of the LV via the surface model. Functional parameters known from other modalities were transferred to the C-arm CT data. The feasibility study on simulated phantom LVs with pathological defects as well as on eight clinical datasets indicate the capability of the presented framework. The dynamic surface model together with the color overlay of the contraction activity in 3-D can provide additional use. The combination of the wall motion analysis with the motion-compensated reconstruction might be of great value to the diagnostic of pathological regions in cardiac interventions. In conclusion, this is the first framework which enables LV wall motion analysis directly in the catheter lab during a cardiac intervention using intra-procedural C-arm CT data.

CHAPTER **4**

Volume-based Cardiac Motion Estimation and Compensated Reconstruction

4.1 Motivation and Clinical Applications 76

4.2 Acquisition and Contrast Protocol 77

4.3 Motion Estimation and Compensation via Registration 77

4.4 Complexity Analysis 93

4.5 Implementation Details and Parameter Setting 95

4.6 Evaluation and Results 99

4.7 First Clinical Patient Data 119

4.8 Challenges 122

4.9 Summary and Conclusions 122

In the previous chapter, the focus was on motion-compensated reconstruction of the left heart ventricle and its wall motion analysis using a surface-based technique. In this chapter, a different problem is addressed, where two or four chambers shall be reconstructed. A three-dimensional cardiac motion-compensated reconstruction of the cardiac chambers is well suited to support the cardiologist during cardiac interventions, for example to guide radio-frequency ablation procedures to cure patients suffering from cardiac arrythmias [De B 13b, Wiel 14]. The goal is to develop a motion estimation and compensation algorithm based on a single sweep scan protocol without surface models to visualize the cardiac chambers. A longer scan and different contrast protocols are necessary to visualize a non-sparse object like the heart chambers, cf. Section 2.7. With the new imaging protocol, the quality of the retrospective ECG-gated reconstructions is increased and these volumes provide the possibility to use them as basis for cardiac motion estimation. Here, three different volume-based cardiac motion estimation approaches are presented utilizing multi-dimensional image registration techniques.

At the beginning of this chapter, the clinical motivation and background is presented in Section 4.1. In Section 4.2, the used single rotation acquisition of the C-arm system and the used contrast protocol are explained in more detail. The three motion estimation approaches using 3-D/(3+N)-D image registration are presented in

Section 4.3. The estimated cardiac motion is then used for a motion-compensated reconstruction using all acquired projection images. In order to compare the different motion estimation techniques, their computational complexity is analysed in Section 4.4. The implementation details and the parameter settings of the experiments for the methods are given in Section 4.5. In Section 4.6, the evaluation strategy for the different datasets is explained and the reconstruction results are presented. In Section 4.7, the preliminary results on a first clinical patient dataset are shown. Section 4.8 explains the challenges and limitations of the presented approaches in clinical practice. The whole chapter ends with a short summary and conclusions in Section 4.9.

Parts of this work have already been published in Müller et al. [Mlle 12a, Mlle 13d, Mlle 14a, Mlle 14b].

4.1 Motivation and Clinical Applications

Most catheter-based cardiac interventions are monitored using fluoroscopic images provided by a flexible angiographic C-arm system. In order to guide the cardiologist in some procedures, pre-interventional acquired US or MRI data are overlayed onto the 2-D acquired X-ray images [Ma 12]. Additionally, C-arm systems provide the ability to perform 3-D imaging. The three-dimensional reconstruction can be overlayed on the interventional 2-D projection images to provide additional support to the cardiologist [Hett 10, Bros 12] directly in the catheter lab without the need for another CT or MRI scan.

In John et al. [John 10], the 3-D reconstruction of the aortic root is used for guidance of a transcatheter aortic valve implantation (TAVI) by overlaying the 3-D reconstruction onto the fluoroscopic images during the deployment of the prosthesis and to measure critical anatomical parameters in 3-D image space. However, this approach is limited to reconstruct the aortic root and cannot visualize the ventricular outflow tract (non-circular aortic annulus), which is also of clinical interest for TAVI procedures [Schu 13].

Up to now, pre-operative four-dimensional echocardiographic volumes are used for wall motion analysis for cardiac resynchronization therapy (CRT) procedures in order to find the optimal lead position [Drin 13]. The incorporation of dynamics allows to visualize new characteristics of a patient's heart. The 3-D C-arm CT reconstruction of the coronary sinus is overlayed onto the 2-D fluoroscopic images and on the 4-D echocardiographic volumes. The multi-modal image fusion is used to identify coronary sinus branches close to the area of the latest mechanical activation in order to place the pacemaker electrode. Three-dimensional C-arm reconstructions of the whole cardiac chambers in various heart states directly in the catheter lab would provide valuable information for the cardiologist, e.g., during CRT procedures. The application of 3-D dynamic echocardiography is not widely spread during all cardiac procedures and C-arm CT imaging allows for an easier use under sterile clinical conditions.

In some clinical procedures, e.g., pulmonary vein isolation and pulmonary artery interventions, standard 3-D reconstructions have proven to be useful, despite the slight motion blur, since these are relatively static structures [Nlke 10, Schw 11]. However, 3-D imaging of valvular structures [John 10] or the ventricles using C-arm CT, is either done by administration of adenosine to slow the heart rate of a patient to a minimum or even stop it for a short time. Alternatively, rapid pacing is applied to increase the heart frequency to prevent the heart from a full contraction [Ecto 09] and to turn the heart beat into a slight jitter. Usually, pacing frequencies of about 220 bpm are used [Daeh 04]. However, this bears a risk of tachycardias and circulatory collapse during the procedure [Ecto 09].

4.2 Acquisition and Contrast Protocol

The imaging protocol used for imaging two or four heart chambers with one sweep of the C-arm system uses slow external pacing either in the right atrium or right ventricle which leads to a controlled but moderate heart beat of the patient. The heart beat is paced to approximately 130 bpm or less to reduce the risk of tachycardias. The overall acquisition time is about 14 s capturing 381 projection images with 30 f/s, and an angular increment of 0.52° degree during one C-arm sweep [De B 13b]. The contrast agent is administered via the pulmonary artery for the two chamber protocol (left atrium and left ventricle) or in the right atrium or vena cava for four chamber imaging. The contrast administration starts before the imaging. This patient specific X-ray delay is determined by a test bolus injection. The time is given by the time that is required for a full saturation of the heart chambers with contrast agent. The animal datasets were acquired in a research laboratory at the University of Leuven, Belgium. The first clinical datasets were provided by the Herz- und Kreislauf Zentrum, Rotenburg an der Fulda, Germany.

4.3 Cardiac Motion Estimation & Compensation via Multi-Dimensional Registration

The cardiac imaging protocol described in Section 4.2, provides the possibility to reconstruct initial volumes for several heart phases from the acquired projection data. An adequate initial image quality is demanded, which allows for the application of a deformable image registration technique for cardiac motion estimation. Thus, in Section 4.3.1, different reconstruction and subsequent enhancement techniques for the initial images are presented. The different initial reconstructed volumes are used for multi-dimensional deformable image registration to estimate the cardiac motion. The different objective functions and optimization techniques for registration are described in Section 4.3.2. In Section 4.3.3, the final image reconstruction is explained. A schematic overview of the individual steps is given in Figure 4.1.

4.3.1 Initial 3-D Volume Generation

All initial image reconstructions are based on the retrospective single sweep ECG-gating as described in Section 2.3.1.

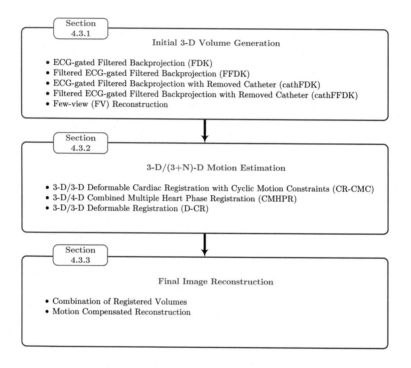

Figure 4.1: Schematic overview of the motion estimation and compensation via 3-D/(3+N)-D registration.

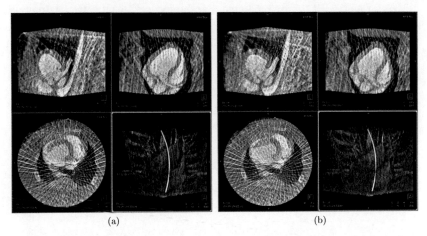

(a)   (b)

Figure 4.2: Example of ECG-gated FDK reconstructions of a porcine model from about 32 projection images at a relative heart phase of (a) 20 % and (b) 80 %. The image data was provided by Prof. Dr. Heidbüchel and Dr. De Buck from the University of Leuven, Belgium.

4.3.1.1   ECG-gated Filtered Backprojection Volume Reconstruction (FDK)

For this approach, the projections are ECG-gated and the volumes are reconstructed with the standard FDK reconstruction algorithm [Feld 84]. The algorithm is explained in Section 2.3.1 and shortly repeated here.

The function $f_{\phi_k}(\boldsymbol{x}, \boldsymbol{s})$ returns the reconstructed object at the 3-D position $\boldsymbol{x}$ and the heart phase $\phi_k \in \{1, \ldots, K\}$, with K denotes a certain number of heart phases to be reconstructed and the vector $\boldsymbol{s} \in \mathbb{R}^{K_s}$ contains all the parameters for the basis functions and the motion model parameters. The heart phase ϕ_k corresponds to a relative heart phase of $\phi \in [0, 1]$. Hence, due to the long acquisition time of the C-arm system, different heart phases can be reconstructed with data from one C-arm rotation by

$$f_{\phi_k}(\boldsymbol{x}, \boldsymbol{s}) = \sum_{i=1}^{N} \lambda(i, \boldsymbol{s}_{\mathrm{ga}}) \cdot h_{\mathrm{FDK}}(i, \boldsymbol{x}), \qquad (4.1)$$

where N is the number of projection images, $\lambda(i, \boldsymbol{s}_{\mathrm{ga}})$ is the view dependent ECG-gated weighting function, $h_{\mathrm{FDK}}(i, \boldsymbol{x})$ denotes the i-th redundancy and filtered projection image, and $\boldsymbol{s}_{\mathrm{ga}} = (\phi_r, w, \vartheta)^{\top}$, cf. Section 2.2.1. For example, if the rotation duration is 14 s and the patient has a heart rate of 120 bpm-130 bpm, and $w \to 0$ (nearest-neighbor gating and only 1 image per heart cycle), 28 projections per heart phase are available. Extending the window width w leads to only slightly increased image quality, since adjacent projections are highly correlated and contain redundant information [Abba 13]. The resulting ECG-gated FDK images are highly corrupted by noise and suffer from severe streak artifacts, as can be seen in Figure 4.2.

4.3.1.2   Filtered ECG-gated Filtered Backprojection Volume Reconstruction (FFDK)

The FDK volumes are additionally filtered by a 3-D bilateral filter [Toma 98] to reduce streak artifacts and eliminate noise. The bilateral filtered volume can be expressed by

$$
f_{\phi_k, f}(\boldsymbol{x}, \boldsymbol{s}) \;=\; \frac{1}{w_p} \sum_{\boldsymbol{x}_v \in \Omega} f_{\phi_k}(\boldsymbol{x}_v, \boldsymbol{s}) \cdot
$$
$$
h_r(||f_{\phi_k}(\boldsymbol{x}_v, \boldsymbol{s}) - f_{\phi_k}(\boldsymbol{x}, \boldsymbol{s})||_2) \cdot h_d(||\boldsymbol{x}_v - \boldsymbol{x}||_2), \tag{4.2}
$$

where Ω defines the region contributing to the filter, and w_p is a normalization factor, according to

$$
w_p = \sum_{\boldsymbol{x}_v \in \Omega} h_r(||f_{\phi_k}(\boldsymbol{x}_v, \boldsymbol{s}) - f_{\phi_k}(\boldsymbol{x}, \boldsymbol{s})||_2) \cdot h_d(||\boldsymbol{x}_v - \boldsymbol{x}||_2). \tag{4.3}
$$

The function h_r describes the similarity in the intensity range of the values, and h_d the spatial closeness using Gaussian filters

$$
h_r(||f_{\phi_k}(\boldsymbol{x}_v, \boldsymbol{s}) - f_{\phi_k}(\boldsymbol{x}, \boldsymbol{s})||_2) \;=\; \exp\left(-\frac{(f_{\phi_k}(\boldsymbol{x}_v, \boldsymbol{s}) - f_{\phi_k}(\boldsymbol{x}, \boldsymbol{s}))^2}{2\sigma_r^2}\right), \tag{4.4}
$$
$$
h_d(||\boldsymbol{x}_v - \boldsymbol{x}||_2) \;=\; \exp\left(-\frac{||\boldsymbol{x}_v - \boldsymbol{x}||_2^2}{2\sigma_d^2}\right). \tag{4.5}
$$

σ_r and σ_d are the adjustable bilateral filter parameters. The edge-preserving bilateral filter can be applied due to the high contrast inside the heart chambers relative to the streak artifacts. However, after filtering, the volumes still exhibit streak artifacts, e.g., caused by catheters and electrodes, see Figure 4.3.

4.3.1.3   ECG-gated Filtered Backprojection Volume Reconstruction with Removed Catheter (cathFDK)

Both approaches from the previous sections suffer not only from noise and undersampling artifacts, but also from artifacts induced by high-density objects like a pigtail catheter or a pacing electrode. Therefore, one way of reducing these artifacts is the removal of these objects from the 2-D projection images. The overall catheter removal procedure is illustrated in Figure 4.4 and described below.

    The high density objects (catheters and pacing electrodes) are identified in the preliminary ECG-gated volumes $f_{\phi_k}(\boldsymbol{x}, \boldsymbol{s})$. The segmentation process of the catheters is restricted to a user defined region of interest (ROI), denoted as $r(\boldsymbol{x})$. For segmentation, the 2-D axial slices of the volumes $f_{\phi_k}(\boldsymbol{x}, \boldsymbol{s})$ are filtered with a 2-D median filter of size 2×2 pixels to reduce noise in the reconstructed volumes. Afterwards, a thresholding operation is applied with a pre-set threshold entered by the user and the segmented pixels are dilated by a circular object with a radius of 1 pixel. Finally, the consistency of the catheter over the slices is automatically checked and completed if necessary. The resulting binary mask images $m_{\phi_k}(\boldsymbol{x}, \boldsymbol{s})$ are forward projected into the

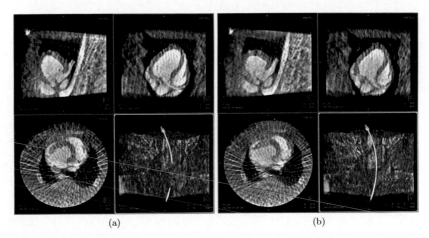

(a)   (b)

Figure 4.3: Example of filtered ECG-gated FDK reconstructions of a porcine model from about 32 projection images at a relative heart phase of (a) 20 % and (b) 80 %. The image data was provided by Prof. Dr. Heidbüchel and Dr. De Buck from the University of Leuven, Belgium.

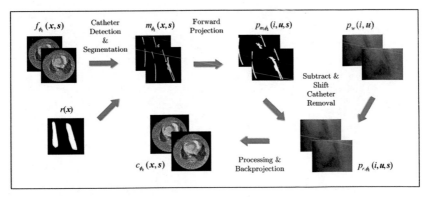

Figure 4.4: Schematic overview of the catheter removal procedure.

2-D projection images, which belong to the same heart phases used for the generation of the preliminary ECG-gated images. As a forward projector, due to its simplicity, a ray casting approach is used as

$$p_{m,\phi_k}(i, \boldsymbol{u}, \boldsymbol{s}) = \max_{\boldsymbol{x} \in L_{i,\boldsymbol{u}}} m_{\phi_k}(\boldsymbol{x}, \boldsymbol{s}), \qquad (4.6)$$

where $L_{i,\boldsymbol{u}} = \{\boldsymbol{x} \in \mathbb{R}^3 | B(i, \boldsymbol{x}) = \boldsymbol{u}\}$ defines the ray of the i-th image intersecting the detector at pixel $\boldsymbol{u}$. Thus, only the set of voxels along the ray $L_{i,\boldsymbol{u}}$ is used. Here, the maximum intensity value is computed along the ray. The 2-D mask images combined with the log-transformed projection images $p_w(i, \boldsymbol{u})$ are used for the catheter removal. In this thesis, a low-frequency-based object masking called Subtract-and-Shift (SaS) is used for the removal of the catheter in the 2-D projection images [Schw 10]. It makes use of the fact that many dense objects do not absorb all incident radiation. Therefore, some remaining anatomical structure is still available within the region overlaid by the object and should be used by an interpolation algorithm. A dense object in the field of view introduces an additive bias or contribution to the projection integral. Therefore, a bias correction similar to bias field correction in MR imaging [Vovk 07] is used:

1. The whole projection image is low-pass filtered: $g_w(i, \boldsymbol{u}) = (p_w \star h_\sigma)(i, \boldsymbol{u})$, where h_σ is a Gaussian kernel with a standard deviation of σ.

2. At every pixel belonging to the object to be removed, the filtered intensity value is subtracted from the measured intensity: $s(i, \boldsymbol{u}) = p_w(i, \boldsymbol{u}) - g_w(i, \boldsymbol{u})$.

3. The intensity values inside the processed region are shifted, such that they match the intensity levels surrounding the region: $\hat{s}(i, \boldsymbol{u}) = s(i, \boldsymbol{u}) + \triangle_I(i, \boldsymbol{u})$, where $\triangle_I(i, \boldsymbol{u})$ is a line-wise interpolated value of the intensity offset $\triangle_I$, before and after the processed region.

Steps (1) and (2) effectively high-pass filter the processed region, removing the low frequency bias field and retaining only the high-frequency content. Since the intensity values after step (2) are centered around 0, they need to be shifted back to the intensity level of their surroundings. This is usually done by adding a mean-preserving value after step (2). Here, a different strategy for the shift step is proposed: a line-wise linear interpolation of $\triangle_I(i, \boldsymbol{u})$. Along an arbitrary line through the processed region, the intensity offsets $\triangle_I$ before and after the region are determined. Then, the intensities along that line, which are inside the region are shifted by a linear interpolation between both offsets to compute $p_{r,\phi_k}(i, \boldsymbol{u}, \boldsymbol{s})$.

The resulting interpolated images $p_{r,\phi_k}(i, \boldsymbol{u}, \boldsymbol{s})$ are used for ECG-gated filtered backprojection reconstruction in order to result in an image $c_{\phi_k}(\boldsymbol{x}, \boldsymbol{s})$ without catheters and electrodes. In Figure 4.5, example reconstructions are presented. It can be seen that the streak artifacts are reduced compared to a standard ECG-gated FDK reconstruction, cf. Figure 4.2.

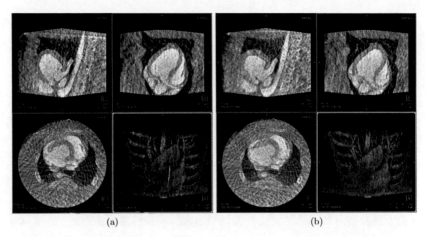

(a)   (b)

Figure 4.5: Example of ECG-gated FDK reconstructions of a porcine model with removed catheter and pacing electrode at a relative heart phase of (a) 20 % and (b) 80 %. The image data was provided by Prof. Dr. Heidbüchel and Dr. De Buck from the University of Leuven, Belgium.

4.3.1.4   Filtered ECG-gated Filtered Backprojection Volume Reconstruction with Removed Catheter (cathFFDK)

The volumes from the previous section still exhibit strong noise. Hence, an additional bilateral filter can be applied, cf. Section 4.3.1.2, resulting in $c_{\phi_k,f}(\boldsymbol{x}, \boldsymbol{s})$. Example reconstructions are shown in Figure 4.6.

4.3.1.5   Few-view Volume Reconstruction (FV)

Additionally, images denoted as $v_{\phi_k}(\boldsymbol{x}, \boldsymbol{s})$ are reconstructed with an iterative few-view reconstruction algorithm that takes the sparse sampling condition into account. Here, the prior image constrained compressed sensing (PICCS) [Chen 08] combined with the improved total variation (iTV) [Rits 11] algorithm is used. Both approaches are described in more detail in Section 2.2.2.2. A brief summary is provided here. An FDK reconstruction with data from a complete short-scan is used as prior volume for the PICCS reconstruction. The objective function is minimized in an alternating manner, i.e. the raw data constraint is minimized in a first step and in the second step the sparsity cost function, which incorporates knowledge of the prior image, is optimized. In order to ensure that the raw data cost function converges to the optimal value and simultaneously ensure that the sparsity constraint converges to a low value, the improved total variation (iTV) is used [Rits 11]. In order to minimize the data truncation artifact, the volume for reconstruction was chosen slightly larger than the field of view. In Figure 4.7, it can be seen that the resulting volumes have minor streak artifacts, but appear to have visually smoother edges than the ECG-gated reconstructions.

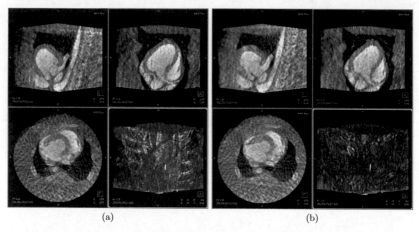

Figure 4.6: Example of filtered ECG-gated FDK reconstructions of a porcine model with removed catheter and pacing electrode at a relative heart phase of (a) 20 % and (b) 80 %. The image data was provided by Prof. Dr. Heidbüchel and Dr. De Buck from the University of Leuven, Belgium.

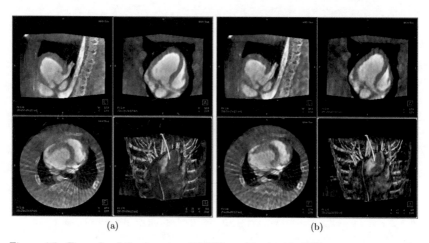

Figure 4.7: Example of the few-view (PICCS combined with iTV) reconstructions of a porcine model at a relative heart phase of (a) 20 % and (b) 80 %. The image data was provided by Prof. Dr. Heidbüchel and Dr. De Buck from the University of Leuven, Belgium.

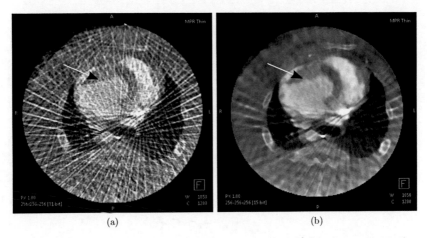

(a)   (b)

Figure 4.8: Comparison of ECG-gated FDK reconstruction and few-view reconstruction. (a) Example of ECG-gated FDK reconstructions at a relative heart phase of 20 %. (b) Example of the few-view (PICCS combined with iTV) reconstructions of a porcine model at a relative heart phase of 20 %. The arrow indicates the smoother endocardial edge. The image data was provided by Prof. Dr. Heidbüchel and Dr. De Buck from the University of Leuven, Belgium.

4.3.2   3-D/(3+N)-D Objective Function & Optimization Strategy

In this part, the three different objective functions and optimization strategies used for cardiac motion estimation are explained in more detail. The first registration technique is an adaption of a motion estimation approach developed for respiratory motion estimation and compensation [Breh 12]. It incorporates cyclic motion constraints into the registration process. Therefore, it is denoted as 3-D/3-D deformable cardiac registration with cyclic motion constraints (CR-CMC). The second approach utilizes a reference image of improved image quality and registers the sum of the FDK volumes to this reference volume. Hence it is called 3-D/4-D combined multiple heart phase registration (CMHPR) approach. The third approach uses a deformable 3-D/3-D registration between a depicted reference volume and all other initial volumes individually. Here, the cardiac motion is represented by a B-spline model. This approach is called 3-D/3-D deformable cardiac registration (D-CR).

4.3.2.1   3-D/3-D Deformable Cardiac Registration with Cyclic Motion Constraints (CR-CMC)

The 3-D/3-D deformable cardiac registration with cyclic motion constraints (CR-CMC) is an adaption of an algorithm presented by Brehm et al. [Breh 12] for respiratory motion estimation and compensation in radiation therapy. In image-guided radiation therapy an additional kV system mounted next to the linear particle accelerator is used for patient positioning. The acquisition time of the system is much longer

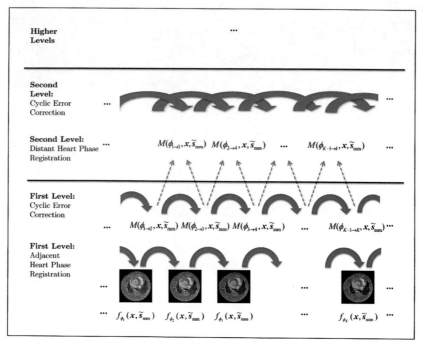

Figure 4.9: Overview of the 3-D/3-D deformable cardiac registration with cyclic motion constraints (CR-CMC).

than the patient's breathing cycle. In the respiratory gated volumes, streak artifacts occur similar to the artifacts induced by ECG-gating. The assumption is made that a motion estimation approach using image registration techniques matches the streaks inside the volumes instead of the anatomical information. To reduce the influence of the streak artifacts on the deformation, cyclic constraints were incorporated into the registration process.

The CR-CMC algorithm comprises mainly a spatial registration and a periodic correction of the motion vector fields between the reconstructed volumes. In Figure 4.9, a scheme of the CR-CMC registration process is illustrated. The details are explained in the following section.

In order to estimate the cardiac motion, a motion model function M needs to be defined. The function M describes the mapping from any heart phase ϕ_j to the heart phase ϕ_k and can be described by

$$M(\phi_{j \to k}, \boldsymbol{x}, \tilde{\boldsymbol{s}}_{\mathrm{mm}}) = \boldsymbol{x} + \tilde{\boldsymbol{s}}_{\mathrm{mm}, \boldsymbol{x}}, \tag{4.7}$$

where $\tilde{\boldsymbol{s}}_{\mathrm{mm}, \boldsymbol{x}} \in \mathbb{R}^3$ denotes the displacement vector at voxel position $\boldsymbol{x}$ and $\tilde{\boldsymbol{s}}_{\mathrm{mm}} \in \mathbb{R}^{\widetilde{K}_{\mathrm{mm}}}$ the motion vector parameters between the reference and the current heart phase. Here, a voxel based motion model is used, where $\widetilde{K}_{\mathrm{mm}} = 3n^3$, with n denoting the side length of the reconstructed volume. The mapping between adjacent volumes can then be defined as

$$f_{\phi_{k+1}}(\boldsymbol{x}, \tilde{\boldsymbol{s}}_{\mathrm{mm}}) = f_{\phi_k}(M(\phi_{k\to k+1}, \boldsymbol{x}, \tilde{\boldsymbol{s}}_{\mathrm{mm}}), \tilde{\boldsymbol{s}}_{\mathrm{mm}}). \tag{4.8}$$

In order to obtain a complete definition of the cardiac motion over the whole scan, the motion needs to be estimated between all heart phases, consequently K times. Hence, the number of parameters $\boldsymbol{s}_{\mathrm{mm}} \in \mathbb{R}^{K_{\mathrm{mm}}}$ is given by $K_{\mathrm{mm}} = K \cdot \tilde{K}_{\mathrm{mm}}$.

The motion model function parameter $\tilde{\boldsymbol{s}}_{\mathrm{mm}}$ between two adjacent heart phases are estimated by deformable image registration. In order to evaluate the proposed algorithm by Brehm et al. [Breh 12] on cardiac C-arm data, the original objective function has been reimplemented. A deformable registration algorithm originally proposed by Thirion et al. [Thir 98] called demon's algorithm is used. Several variants of the demon's algorithm have been proposed depending on the computation of the demon's forces. Here, a diffeomorphic demon's algorithm [Verc 09] using symmetric forces [Wang 05] is used with an adaptive step width control [Cach 99] and a viscous fluid-like and an elastic-like appearance [Penn 99]. Since the demon's algorithm is based on optical flow and - because of this - intensity measurements, the gray scale values between the initial volumes are normalized by histogram matching [Nyul 00]. The reconstructions are afterwards filtered with a bilateral filter as presented in Section 4.3.1.2. Using the assumption of a cyclic cardiac motion, a phase index $K + j$ is synonymous with the index j, i.e. all phase indices are to be understood by a modulo operation. Accordingly, the non-commutative concatenation $\prod$ of several motion vector functions is denoted as

$$\prod_{k=1}^{K} M(\phi_{k\to k+1}, \boldsymbol{x}, \tilde{\boldsymbol{s}}_{\mathrm{mm}}) = M(\phi_{1\to 2}, \boldsymbol{x}, \tilde{\boldsymbol{s}}_{\mathrm{mm}}) \circ \ldots$$
$$\ldots M(\phi_{2\to 3}, \boldsymbol{x}, \tilde{\boldsymbol{s}}_{\mathrm{mm}}) \circ \ldots \circ M(\phi_{K\to 1}, \boldsymbol{x}, \tilde{\boldsymbol{s}}_{\mathrm{mm}}). \tag{4.9}$$

Now, the assumption of cyclic motion is that the non-commutative concatenation of the resulting motion vector functions, between all heart phases, results in the identity function id. The deviation of the concatenation of the MVFs from the identity function for one heart phase is denoted as

$$E_k = (\prod_{j=k}^{K+k-1} M(\phi_{j\to j+1}, \boldsymbol{x}, \tilde{\boldsymbol{s}}_{\mathrm{mm}})) - \mathrm{id}. \tag{4.10}$$

The overall motion error E is then defined as

$$E = \sum_{k=1}^{K} \|E_k\|_2^2. \tag{4.11}$$

The registration algorithm needs to keep the error E sufficiently small during estimation. In order to correct for the error E, a correction term is defined, such that the error induced by each motion function contributes equally to the error. For each heart phase j, its motion model needs to be updated for all K errors E_k according to

$$\widetilde{M}(\phi_{j\to j+1}, \boldsymbol{x}, \tilde{\boldsymbol{s}}_{\mathrm{mm}}) = \begin{cases} M(\phi_{j\to j+1}, \boldsymbol{x}, \tilde{\boldsymbol{s}}_{\mathrm{mm}}) - \frac{E_k}{K} & j = k \\ M(\phi_{j\to j+1}, \boldsymbol{x}, \tilde{\boldsymbol{s}}_{\mathrm{mm}}) - \frac{E_k \circ \prod_{l=k}^{j-1} M(\phi_{l\to l+1}, \boldsymbol{x}, \tilde{\boldsymbol{s}}_{\mathrm{mm}})}{K} & j \neq k \end{cases} \tag{4.12}$$

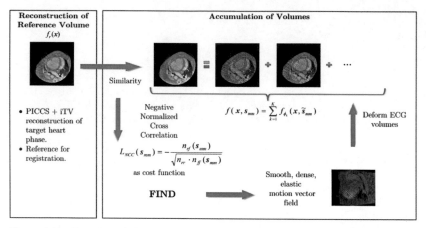

Figure 4.10: Overview of the combined multiple heart phase registration (CMHPR) approach.

Up to now, only adjacent heart phases are registered to each other, but the motion compensation also requires mappings between non-adjacent phases. Consequently, a hierarchical registration is used to register non-adjacent phases with the previously estimated motion vector fields as initialization. On each level, the spatial registration and the motion error correction is performed. A more detailed explanation of the algorithm can be found in Brehm et al. [Breh 12, Breh 13].

4.3.2.2 3-D/4-D Combined Multiple Heart Phase Registration (CMHPR)

For the 3-D/4-D combined multiple heart phase registration (CMHPR) approach, in order to estimate the cardiac motion, one heart phase needs to be selected as reference phase. A sum volume $f(\boldsymbol{x}, \boldsymbol{s}_{\mathrm{mm}})$ is defined consisting of the deformed ECG-gated volumes $f_{\phi_k}(\boldsymbol{x}, \boldsymbol{s}_{\mathrm{mm}})$ with motion vector parameter $\tilde{\boldsymbol{s}}_{\mathrm{mm}} \in \mathbb{R}^{\widetilde{K}_{\mathrm{mm}}}$ at heart phase ϕ_k and location $\boldsymbol{x}$

$$f(\boldsymbol{x}, \boldsymbol{s}_{\mathrm{mm}}) = \sum_{k=1}^{K} f_{\phi_k}(\boldsymbol{x}, \tilde{\boldsymbol{s}}_{\mathrm{mm}}). \qquad (4.13)$$

For this approach, a voxel-based motion vector field is used, consequently $\widetilde{K}_{\mathrm{mm}} = 3n^3$, with n denoting the side length of the reconstructed volume. The motion vector parameter $\boldsymbol{s}_{\mathrm{mm}} \in \mathbb{R}^{K_{\mathrm{mm}}}$ contains the motion parameters for all heart phases, thus, $K_{\mathrm{mm}} = K \widetilde{K}_{\mathrm{mm}}$. Here, it is assumed that the reference heart phase is also represented in the initial ECG-gated reconstructions, but it is not necessarily required. The motion model function M describes the mapping from a reference phase ϕ_r to the current heart phase ϕ_k and is described by

$$M(\phi_{r \to k}, \boldsymbol{x}, \dot{\boldsymbol{s}}_{\mathrm{mm}}) = \boldsymbol{x} + \tilde{\boldsymbol{s}}_{\mathrm{mm}, \boldsymbol{x}}. \qquad (4.14)$$

The 4-D motion vector field is then derived by optimizing an objective function $\mathcal{L}_{NCC}(\boldsymbol{s}_{\text{mm}})$ so that the negative normalized cross correlation (NCC) between the sum volume $f(\boldsymbol{x}, \boldsymbol{s}_{\text{mm}})$ and a reference volume $f_r(\boldsymbol{x})$ is minimized. In this thesis, exemplarily the few-view reconstruction is used to generate the reference volume $f_r(\boldsymbol{x}) = v_{\phi_k}(\boldsymbol{x}, \boldsymbol{s})$. The assumption is that the few-view reconstruction delineates the borders and edges of the endocardium and that the sum of the ECG-gated reconstructions features less streak artifacts compared to the single ECG-gated reconstructions. The negative NCC metric ranges between $[-1, 1]$. In order to define a dissimilarity measure, the negative correlation is considered. Therefore, a value of -1 indicates a perfect positive linear relationship, a value of +1 a perfect negative linear relationship and values close to zero show no linear correlation between the volumes. The definition of the negative NCC [Russ 03, Penn 98] combined with the computational formula for the variance [Knut 98] is given by

$$\hat{\boldsymbol{s}}_{\text{mm}} = \arg\min_{\boldsymbol{s}_{\text{mm}}} \mathcal{L}_{NCC}(\boldsymbol{s}_{\text{mm}}), \qquad \text{with} \tag{4.15}$$

$$\mathcal{L}_{NCC}(\boldsymbol{s}_{\text{mm}}) = -\frac{n_{rf}(\boldsymbol{s}_{\text{mm}})}{\sqrt{n_{rr} \cdot n_{ff}(\boldsymbol{s}_{\text{mm}})}}, \qquad \text{where} \tag{4.16}$$

$$n_r = \sum_{\boldsymbol{x} \in \Omega} f_r(\boldsymbol{x}) \tag{4.17}$$

$$n_f(\boldsymbol{s}_{\text{mm}}) = \sum_{\boldsymbol{x} \in \Omega} f(\boldsymbol{x}, \boldsymbol{s}_{\text{mm}}) \tag{4.18}$$

$$n_{rr} = \sum_{\boldsymbol{x} \in \Omega} f_r(\boldsymbol{x})^2 - \frac{1}{|\Omega|} n_r^2 \tag{4.19}$$

$$n_{ff}(\boldsymbol{s}_{\text{mm}}) = \sum_{\boldsymbol{x} \in \Omega} f(\boldsymbol{x}, \boldsymbol{s}_{\text{mm}})^2 - \frac{1}{|\Omega|} n_f(\boldsymbol{s}_{\text{mm}})^2 \tag{4.20}$$

$$n_{rf}(\boldsymbol{s}_{\text{mm}}) = \sum_{\boldsymbol{x} \in \Omega} f_r(\boldsymbol{x}) f(\boldsymbol{x}, \boldsymbol{s}_{\text{mm}}) - \frac{1}{|\Omega|} n_r \cdot n_f(\boldsymbol{s}_{\text{mm}}). \tag{4.21}$$

The objective function is minimized by a gradient based quasi-Newton method, a so called limited-memory Broyden-Fletcher-Goldfarb-Shanno optimizer (L-BFGS) [Flet 70]. Usually, the quasi-Newton based methods converge in fewer iterations than gradient descent optimizers, but have a higher cost per iteration evaluation. For the optimization, the derivative of the objective function with respect to the motion vector for every heart phase and at every voxel is required. It can be computed as

$$\frac{\partial \mathcal{L}_{NCC}(\boldsymbol{s}_{\text{mm}})}{\partial \boldsymbol{s}_{\text{mm},x}} = -\left(\frac{1}{\sqrt{n_{rr} \cdot n_{ff}(\boldsymbol{s}_{\text{mm}})}} \frac{\partial n_{rf}(\boldsymbol{s}_{\text{mm}})}{\partial \boldsymbol{s}_{\text{mm},x}} - \frac{n_{rf}(\boldsymbol{s}_{\text{mm}}) \cdot n_{rr}}{2\sqrt{(n_{rr} \cdot n_{ff}(\boldsymbol{s}_{\text{mm}}))^3}} \frac{\partial n_{ff}(\boldsymbol{s}_{\text{mm}})}{\partial \boldsymbol{s}_{\text{mm},x}} \right), \tag{4.22}$$

where the remaining components are given by

$$\frac{\partial n_{rf}(\boldsymbol{s}_{\text{mm}})}{\partial \boldsymbol{s}_{\text{mm},x}} = \left(f_r(\boldsymbol{x}) - \frac{n_r}{|\Omega|} \right) \frac{\partial f(\boldsymbol{x}, \boldsymbol{s}_{\text{mm}})}{\partial \boldsymbol{s}_{\text{mm},x}} \tag{4.23}$$

and

$$\frac{\partial n_{ff}(s_{\text{mm}})}{\partial s_{\text{mm},x}} = 2 \left(f(x, s_{\text{mm}}) - \frac{n_f(s_{\text{mm}})}{|\Omega|} \right) \frac{\partial f(x, s_{\text{mm}})}{\partial s_{\text{mm},x}}. \qquad (4.24)$$

Finally, putting all components together the derivative of the objective function is given as

$$\begin{aligned}
\frac{\partial \mathcal{L}_{NCC}(s_{\text{mm}})}{\partial s_{\text{mm},x}} &= -\kappa(x, s_{\text{mm}}) \cdot \frac{\partial f(x, s_{\text{mm}})}{\partial s_{\text{mm},x}} \\
&= -\kappa(x, s_{\text{mm}}) \cdot \frac{\partial f_{\phi_k}(x, s_{\text{mm}})}{\partial s_{\text{mm},x}}, \qquad (4.25)
\end{aligned}$$

where

$$\begin{aligned}
\kappa(x, s_{\text{mm}}) &= \frac{1}{\sqrt{n_{rr} \cdot n_{ff}(s_{\text{mm}})}} \left(\left(f_r(x) - \frac{n_r}{|\Omega|} \right) - \right. \\
&\left. \frac{n_{rf}(s_{\text{mm}})}{n_{ff}(s_{\text{mm}})} \left(f(x, s_{\text{mm}}) - \frac{n_f(s_{\text{mm}})}{|\Omega|} \right) \right). \qquad (4.26)
\end{aligned}$$

In order to guarantee a smooth motion vector field, a spatial and temporal approximative recursive Gaussian filter (Deriche filter) is applied to the 4-D motion vector gradient. Additionally, the same approximative spatial recursive Gaussian filter is also applied to the gradient weighting term $\kappa(x, s_{\text{mm}})$ [Deri 87, Deri 93, Deri 90].

4.3.2.3 3-D/3-D Deformable Cardiac Registration (D-CR)

For the 3-D/3-D deformable registration approach (D-CR), in order to estimate the cardiac motion, again one heart phase needs to be selected as reference phase. The corresponding volume is called reference volume and all other volumes are registered pairwise to the reference volume. Here, the registration is carried out between all initial volumes, presented in Section 4.3.1. The reference volume is denoted as $f_r(x)$ and the volumes registered to the reference volume are denoted as template volumes $f_{T,\phi_k}(x, s)$.

The deformable registration is based on a uniform cubic B-spline representation. The use of a B-spline motion model for representation of cardiac motion is very popular in literature [Shec 03, Blon 06, Hans 09, Rohk 10b]. A three-dimensional B-spline is modeled as 3-D tensor product of 1-D B-splines, hence, a number of $C_s \times C_s \times C_s$ control points is placed uniformly in the spatial domain at the 3-D location $l \in \mathbb{R}^3$. The order of the used B-splines is denoted with S_o. Every control point ows its own displacement vector, defining the number of motion model parameters $\widetilde{K}_{\text{mm}} = 3(C_s + S_o)^3$, and $\tilde{s}_{\text{mm}} \in \mathbb{R}^{\widetilde{K}_{\text{mm}}}$ is a linearized version of the control point displacement vectors. The motion model function $M(\phi_{r \to k}, x, \tilde{s}_{\text{mm}})$ between the reference heart phase and the current heart phase is defined by a linear combination of the control point displacement vectors

$$M(\phi_{r \to k}, x, \tilde{s}_{\text{mm}}) = x + \sum_l B_{l_1}(x_1) B_{l_2}(x_2) B_{l_3}(x_3) \tilde{s}_{\text{mm},l}, \qquad (4.27)$$

where B_{l_1}, B_{l_2}, and B_{l_3} denote the B-spline basis functions [Unse 99] and $\tilde{s}_{\text{mm},l}$ defines the displacement vector at the 3-D location l belonging to a certain control point.

The motion vector field is derived by optimizing the objective function $\mathcal{L}_{NCC}(\tilde{s}_{\text{mm}})$ such that the negative normalized cross correlation (NCC) between the template volume $f_{T,\phi_k}(x, \tilde{s}_{\text{mm}})$ and the reference volume $f_r(x)$ is minimized. The objective function is similar to Section 4.3.2.2, except that the volumes are registered individually to the reference volume and the motion model parameters $\tilde{s}_{\text{mm}}$ have a smaller dimension. For the objective function, a value of -1 indicates a perfect positive linear relationship, a value of +1 a perfect negative linear relationship and values close to zero show no linear correlation between the reconstructions. The definition of the negative NCC is given as

$$\hat{s}_{\text{mm}} = \underset{\tilde{s}_{\text{mm}}}{\arg\min}\, \mathcal{L}_{NCC}(\tilde{s}_{\text{mm}}), \qquad \text{with} \qquad (4.28)$$

$$\mathcal{L}_{NCC}(\tilde{s}_{\text{mm}}) = -\frac{n_{rT}(\tilde{s}_{\text{mm}})}{\sqrt{n_{rr} \cdot n_{TT}(\tilde{s}_{\text{mm}})}}, \qquad \text{where} \qquad (4.29)$$

$$n_r = \sum_{x \in \Omega} f_r(x) \qquad (4.30)$$

$$n_T(\tilde{s}_{\text{mm}}) = \sum_{x \in \Omega} f_{T,\phi_k}(x, \tilde{s}_{\text{mm}}) \qquad (4.31)$$

$$n_{rr} = \sum_{x \in \Omega} f_r(x)^2 - \frac{1}{|\Omega|}n_r^2 \qquad (4.32)$$

$$n_{TT}(\tilde{s}_{\text{mm}}) = \sum_{x \in \Omega} f_{T,\phi_k}(x, \tilde{s}_{\text{mm}})^2 - \frac{1}{|\Omega|}n_T(\tilde{s}_{\text{mm}})^2 \qquad (4.33)$$

$$n_{rT}(\tilde{s}_{\text{mm}}) = \sum_{x \in \Omega} f_r(x) f_{T,\phi_k}(x, \tilde{s}_{\text{mm}}) - \frac{1}{|\Omega|}n_r \cdot n_T(\tilde{s}_{\text{mm}}). \qquad (4.34)$$

The optimization is done using an adaptive stochastic gradient descent optimizer [Klei 09]. For the optimization, the derivative of the objective function with respect to the motion vector for every heart phase and at every spline control point l is required. The derivative is given as

$$\frac{\partial \mathcal{L}_{NCC}(\tilde{s}_{\text{mm}})}{\partial \tilde{s}_{\text{mm},l}} = -\left(\frac{1}{\sqrt{n_{rr} \cdot n_{TT}(\tilde{s}_{\text{mm}})}} \frac{\partial n_{rT}(\tilde{s}_{\text{mm}})}{\partial \tilde{s}_{\text{mm},l}} - \right.$$
$$\left. \frac{n_{rT}(\tilde{s}_{\text{mm}}) \cdot n_{rr}}{2\sqrt{(n_{rr} \cdot n_{TT}(\tilde{s}_{\text{mm}}))^3}} \frac{\partial n_{TT}(s)}{\partial \tilde{s}_{\text{mm},l}} \right), \qquad (4.35)$$

where the remaining components are given by

$$\frac{\partial n_{rT}(\tilde{s}_{\text{mm}})}{\partial \tilde{s}_{\text{mm},l}} = \left(f_r(x) - \frac{n_r}{|\Omega|} \right) \frac{\partial f_{T,\phi_k}(x, \tilde{s}_{\text{mm}})}{\partial \tilde{s}_{\text{mm},l}} \qquad (4.36)$$

and

$$\frac{\partial n_{TT}(\tilde{s}_{\text{mm}})}{\partial \tilde{s}_{\text{mm},l}} = 2\left(f_{T,\phi_k}(x, \tilde{s}_{\text{mm}}) - \frac{n_T(\tilde{s}_{\text{mm}})}{|\Omega|} \right) \frac{\partial f_{T,\phi_k}(x, \tilde{s}_{\text{mm}})}{\partial \tilde{s}_{\text{mm},l}}. \qquad (4.37)$$

Finally, putting all components together we arrive at the derivative of the objective function

$$\frac{\partial \mathcal{L}_{NCC}(\tilde{\boldsymbol{s}}_{\mathrm{mm}})}{\partial \tilde{\boldsymbol{s}}_{\mathrm{mm},l}} = -\kappa(\boldsymbol{x}, \tilde{\boldsymbol{s}}_{\mathrm{mm}}) \cdot \frac{\partial f_{T,\phi_k}(\boldsymbol{x}, \tilde{\boldsymbol{s}}_{\mathrm{mm}})}{\partial \tilde{\boldsymbol{s}}_{\mathrm{mm},l}} \tag{4.38}$$

where

$$\kappa(\boldsymbol{x}, \tilde{\boldsymbol{s}}_{\mathrm{mm}}) = \frac{1}{\sqrt{n_{rr} \cdot n_{TT}(\tilde{\boldsymbol{s}}_{\mathrm{mm}})}} \left(\left(f_r(\boldsymbol{x}) - \frac{n_r}{|\Omega|} \right) - \frac{n_{rT}(\tilde{\boldsymbol{s}}_{\mathrm{mm}})}{n_{TT}(\tilde{\boldsymbol{s}}_{\mathrm{mm}})} \left(f_{T,\phi_k}(\boldsymbol{x}, \tilde{\boldsymbol{s}}_{\mathrm{mm}}) - \frac{n_T(\tilde{\boldsymbol{s}}_{\mathrm{mm}})}{|\Omega|} \right) \right). \tag{4.39}$$

In order to obtain a complete cardiac motion field over the whole scan, the motion needs to be estimated between the reference heart phase ϕ_r and the remaining $K-1$ heart phases. Therefore, the dimension of the motion vector $\boldsymbol{s}_{\mathrm{mm}} \in \mathbb{R}^{K_{\mathrm{mm}}}$ results in $K_{\mathrm{mm}} = (K-1) \cdot \widetilde{K}_{\mathrm{mm}}$.

4.3.3 Final Image Reconstruction

The final step to compute the final reconstructed image is either the combination of the deformed 3-D volumes or a motion-compensated reconstruction integrating the estimated motion.

4.3.3.1 Combination of Registered Volumes

For the CMHPR approach, presented in Section 4.3.2.2, the 3-D ECG-gated volumes are already deformed during the registration process in order to fit to the reference volume. Hence, the final volume is already the sum volume denoted as CMHPR reconstruction.

4.3.3.2 Motion Compensated Reconstruction

For final motion-compensated image reconstruction, the estimated motion is integrated into the backprojection step of the FDK algorithm [Gran 02, Schf 06]. The same approach as in Section 2.5.2.2 is used, by integrating the 3-D motion vector fields into the reconstruction. The motion model function $M(\phi_k, \boldsymbol{x}, \boldsymbol{s}_{\mathrm{mm}})$ between all heart phases and the reference heart phase is estimated by the previously presented methods, cf. Section 4.3.2. For every projection image i the assignment to a heart phase ϕ_k is known, cf. Section 3.3.3. If no motion vector field was estimated for the current heart phase, a linear interpolation between neighboring heart phases is sufficient [Prmm 09a]. Therefore, the motion model function $M(i, \boldsymbol{x}, \boldsymbol{s}_{\mathrm{mm}})$ providing a motion vector field is incorporated into a voxel-driven filtered backprojection reconstruction algorithm. The motion correction is applied during the backprojection step by shifting the voxel $\boldsymbol{x}$ to be reconstructed according to the motion function M.

The motion-compensated reconstruction of the cyclic registration is denoted with CR-CMC. The resulting motion-compensated volume for the CMHPR is denoted as CMHPR-MC. The motion-compensated volumes for the D-CR algorithm are denoted by the type of the initial ECG-gated volume reconstruction with added MC for motion-compensation (FDK-MC, FFDK-MC, FV-MC, cathFDK-MC and cathFFDK-MC).

4.4   Complexity Analysis

The computational complexity of the presented motion estimation techniques is described in the following sections.

4.4.1   Initial 3-D Volume Generation

The five approaches for computation of initial images (Section 4.3.1) have different computational complexity. All of them require a backprojection step and some of them an additional forward projection step. The backprojection as well as the forward projection is implemented on a GPU. As a forward projector a ray tracing approach is utilized due to its simplicity and wide-spread use [Sche 11]. The side length of the 3-D volume is denoted as n, the side length of a 2-D projection with m and the number of projections with N. Hence, the complexity of the backprojection-based reconstruction is given as $\mathcal{O}(N\,n^3)$. The generation of the forward projection requires casting a ray from all pixels of all projection images through the volume, resulting in a complexity of $\mathcal{O}(N\,m^2\,n)$.

Therefore, for the FDK reconstruction, the backprojection step is the most time-consuming part with a complexity of $\mathcal{O}(N\,n^3)$. The FFDK utilizes the FDK and additionally performs a filtering step. The used bilateral filter is implemented in a straightforward manner on the GPU and has a complexity of $\mathcal{O}(n^3\,r_f^3)$, where r_f denotes the filter size, which was chosen to be $r_f = 5$. Assuming that $r_f^3 \ll N$, the overall complexity is $\mathcal{O}(N\,n^3)$. In order to generate the cathFDK volumes, two full backprojection steps need to be performed on the GPU each with a complexity of $\mathcal{O}(N\,n^3)$. Afterwards, the most complex part of the segmentation step is the forward projection step with $\mathcal{O}(N\,m^2\,n)$. In total, only two backprojection and one forward projection steps are necessary and the interpolation scheme is of less computational effort, resulting in $\mathcal{O}(N\,n^3)$ under the assumption that $n \approx m$. The cathFFDK approach requires an additional filtering step with $\mathcal{O}(n^3\,r_f^3)$, resulting in the overall complexity of $\mathcal{O}(N\,n^3)$. The FV optimization consists of an iterative optimization scheme for the data consistency term, therefore, several forward and backprojection steps are required. Under the assumption that $n \approx m$, the overall complexity results in $\mathcal{O}(D\,N\,n^3)$, with D denoting the number of data consistency iterations. Each iteration of the FV cost function requires several evaluations of the cost function. The gradient descent search with G iterations for the optimal candidates from the exhaustive search exhibits a complexity of $\mathcal{O}(G\,n^3)$. Therefore, the complexity of the FV objective function results in $\mathcal{O}(F\,G\,n^3)$, with F denoting the number of objective function iterations. The data consistency term and the optimization routine are enclosed by an outer iteration loop and are computed for O iterations. Assuming that $O \approx F \approx D$, the overall complexity is $\mathcal{O}(D^2\,N\,n^3) + \mathcal{O}(D^2\,G\,n^3)$. The overall resulting complexities of the algorithms are presented in Table 4.1.

	FDK	FFDK	cathFDK	cathFFDK	FV
$\mathcal{O}$-calc.	$\mathcal{O}(N\,n^3)$	$\mathcal{O}(N\,n^3)$	$\mathcal{O}(N\,n^3)$	$\mathcal{O}(N\,n^3)$	$\mathcal{O}(D^2\,N\,n^3) + \mathcal{O}(D^2\,G\,n^3)$

Table 4.1: Complexity analysis of the different initial image reconstruction algorithms.

	CR-CMC	CMHPR	D-CR
$\mathcal{O}$-calc.	$\mathcal{O}(H\,T\,S_L\,W\,K^2\,n^3)$	$\mathcal{O}(W\,K\,n^3)$	$\mathcal{O}(S_L\,W\,(K-1)\,(C_s+3)^3)$

Table 4.2: Complexity analysis of the different motion estimation algorithms.

4.4.2   3-D/(3+N)-D Registration

An overview of the complexity of the different cardiac motion estimation algorithms is given in Table 4.2. A more detailed analysis is given in the following sections.

4.4.2.1   CR-CMC

For the 3-D/3-D cardiac registration with cyclic constraints (CR-CMC), the same number of motion parameters as voxels are necessary. Accordingly, the number of parameters is given as $s_{\mathrm{mm}} \in \mathbb{R}^{K_{\mathrm{mm}}=K\cdot 3n^3}$, with n denoting the side length of the volume and K the number of heart phases. For estimation of the spatial transformation that means updating the demon's function, a number of S_L multi-resolution scales are defined, and on each stage a number of W iterations are performed. In every iteration, an update of the demon's registration function is required, i.e. an update of the motion vector parameters with additional exponential filtering [Verc 09]. This results in a comprehensive complexity of $\mathcal{O}(S_L\,W\,K\,n^3)$. The iterative cyclic motion correction requires an update of each motion parameter for multiple times T, thus, it results in a complexity of $\mathcal{O}(T\,S_L\,W\,K\,n^3)$. The spatial transformation estimation and the cyclic motion correction can be performed H times on each level and hierarchical with $L = K - 1$ levels. Therefore, the overall resulting complexity is

$$\mathcal{O}(H\,T\,S_L\,W\,K^2\,n^3).$$

4.4.2.2   CMHPR

For the 3-D/4-D combined multiple heart phase registration (CMHPR), the same number of motion parameters as voxels are required. The number of parameters is therefore given as $s_{\mathrm{mm}} \in \mathbb{R}^{K_{\mathrm{mm}}=K\cdot 3n^3}$, with n denoting the side length of the volume and K the number of heart phases. Due to memory limitations when using a quasi-Newton optimizer and to reduce computation time, the motion vector field was first computed on downsampled volumes with a side length of $0.5\,n$ and upsampled onto the final reconstructed volume size by cubic spline interpolation.

For minimization of the objective function, a number of W iterations of the L-BFGS optimizer are performed. In every iteration, the objective function and its derivative with respect to the motion parameters needs to be evaluated. Resulting in a complexity of $\mathcal{O}(W\,K\,n^3)$. The filtering for κ and the motion vector parameters

s_{mm} result in a complexity independent of the filter size [Deri 90]. Therefore, the comprehensive complexity of the CMHPR algorithm is

$$\mathcal{O}(W\,K\,n^3).$$

4.4.2.3   D-CR

For the D-CR, the motion model function is defined by deformable B-splines. Therefore, the number of parameters is given as $s_{\mathrm{mm}} \in \mathbb{R}^{K_{\mathrm{mm}}}$, where $K_{\mathrm{mm}} = (K-1) \cdot 3(C_s + S_o)^3$, the number of spline control points is given as C_s, S_o denotes the order of the used B-spline, and K denotes the number of heart phases. In this thesis, cubic B-splines are used and, hence, the $S_o = 3$, consequently $s_{\mathrm{mm}} \in \mathbb{R}^{K_{\mathrm{mm}}=(K-1)\cdot 3(C_s+3)^3}$. A number of S_L multi-resolution scales are defined, and on each stage a number of W iterations of the adaptive stochastic gradient descent optimizer needs to be performed. In every iteration, the objective function and its derivative with respect to the motion parameters needs to be computed. This results in a overall complexity of

$$\mathcal{O}(S_L\,W\,(K-1)\,(C_s+3)^3).$$

4.4.3   Motion-compensated Reconstruction

The final step of all presented motion estimation approaches is the motion-compensated reconstruction step. This step results in a complexity of

$$\mathcal{O}(N\,n^3).$$

4.5   Implementation Details and Parameter Setting

This section covers the necessary algorithmic details for implementation and all required parameter settings.

4.5.1   Initial 3-D Volume Generation

For the different initial volume reconstructions, different parameters need to be set.

4.5.1.1   ECG-gating Parameter Setting

The ECG-gating parameters $s_{\mathrm{ga}} = (\phi_r, w, \vartheta)^T$ need to be set for the initial volume reconstruction. In this thesis, due to the acquisition protocol explained in Section 4.2, a rectangular gating function, with $\vartheta = 0$ and of minimal width $w \to 0$, i.e. only one view per heart cycle is considered. In total, K volumes, with $k = 1,\dots,K$ at specific heart phases are reconstructed. Every heart phase ϕ_k corresponds to a relative heart phase ϕ between $[0,1]$ defined between two successive R-peaks. The number of heart phases K is dependent on the acquisition duration and heart frequency of the patient.

4.5.1.2   Bilateral Filter Setting

The parameters of the bilateral filter were set to $\sigma_r = 100$ HU, $\sigma_d = 1$ voxel and the filter kernel size was set to 5. It should be mentioned that if the acquisition scenario changes, these values also need to be adapted.

4.5.1.3   Few-view Parameter Setting

The weighting parameter α for the PICCS algorithm was set to 0.5, which is the upper bound of the optimal range from 0.4 to 0.5, as evaluated in [Thri 12b]. The relaxation parameter β for the data fidelity optimization was set to 0.8 and the iTV parameter ω to 0.8 as in the original paper [Rits 10]. A number of $D = 4$ data consistency, $F = 10$ few-view objective function iterations were set. The whole optimization scheme was stopped when the data error improvement in the subsequent iterations fell below 10 %. A gradient descent optimizer with an adaptive line search was used for minimization of the objective function.

4.5.2   3-D/(3+N)-D Registration

In this section, the different parameter settings for the objective function optimizations to estimate the cardiac motion are presented.

4.5.2.1   CR-CMC

For the CR-CMC approach, first parameters need to be set for the spatial transformation estimation with the diffeomorphic demon's algorithm. Therefore, a multi-scale approach was used with $S_L = 3$ scales. In this thesis, an available implementation of the diffeomorphic demon's inside the Insight Segmentation and RegistrationToolkit[1] was used. On each pyramid level, a number of $W = 20$ iterations were set. The standard deviations of the viscous fluid-like Gaussian convolution kernel G_{pre} and of the elastic like appearance Gaussian kernel G_{post} of the diffeomorphic demon's registration [Penn 99] were set to 1.0 according to Wang et al. [Wang 05]. The maximum step length of the demon's force was set to 2, as described Vercauteren et al. [Verc 07]. The maximal intensity difference or error for numerical stability was set to 0.01. The overall cyclic motion correction was performed once on each level ($T = 1$). The spatial registration and cyclic motion correction on each level were repeated heuristically $H = 3$ times. The number of levels L is determined by the number of heart phases $L = K - 1$. The initial motion vectors between the adjacent heart phase volumes were set to zero.

4.5.2.2   CMHPR Parameter Setting

As previously mentioned, due to memory limitations when using a quasi-Newton optimizer and to reduce computation time, the motion vector field was first computed on downsampled volumes at a resolution of 128^3 voxels and upsampled onto the final reconstructed volume size by cubic spline interpolation. The initial motion vector

---

[1]http://www.itk.org/

field was set to zero in all dimensions. The Deriche filter parameter α_D for spatial filtering was heuristically set to 0.94 and for temporal filtering to 2.12, i.e. a stronger smoothing in spatial than in temporal direction. The L-BFGS optimizer of the VNL[2] numerics library delivered with the Insight Segmentation and Registration Toolkit (ITK)[1] was used for the optimization. The optimization parameters and termination criteria of the L-BFGS algorithm are set as follows: the cost function convergence factor is set to $1 \cdot 10^5$, the projected gradient tolerance is set to $1 \cdot 10^{-30}$, the maximum number of function evaluations is set to 200, the maximum number of variable metric corrections is set to a value of 5. The optimization procedure was performed until the termination criterion was reached. The number of iterations is implicitly given by the number of function evaluations. During the line search of the gradient update, the objective function is evaluated more than once if we are close to a minimum, hence, less iterations are performed. In order to restrict the motion vector field to a local area where the heart motion is expected, a local motion mask enforces zero motion outside the defined local area. In this first approach the mask volume defining Ω is generated manually by the user.

Algorithm 4.1: Combined Multiple Heart Phase Registration (CMHPR).

Input: reference volume $f_r(\boldsymbol{x})$, ECG-gating parameter vector
$\boldsymbol{s}_{\mathrm{ga}} = (\phi_r, w, \vartheta)^T$, mask region Ω, multi-resolution levels S_L

Output: $\boldsymbol{s}_{\mathrm{mm}}$ (contains all $\tilde{\boldsymbol{s}}_{\mathrm{mm}}$)

      // Step 1: Compute initial ECG-gated volumes according to
          Equation 2.20

1 $\tilde{\boldsymbol{s}}_{\mathrm{mm}} = 0$

2 $f_{\phi_k}(\boldsymbol{x}, \tilde{\boldsymbol{s}}_{\mathrm{mm}}) = \sum_{i=1}^{N} \lambda(i, \boldsymbol{s}_{\mathrm{ga}}) \cdot h_{\mathrm{FDK}}(i, \boldsymbol{x})$
      // Step 2: Multi-resolution optimization

3 $\boldsymbol{s}_{\mathrm{mm}} = 0$

4 **for** $s \leftarrow 1$ **to** S_L **do**

5   Compute downsampled volumes $f_r(\boldsymbol{x})$, $f_{\phi_k}(\boldsymbol{x}, \tilde{\boldsymbol{s}}_{\mathrm{mm}})$
         // Step 3: start optimization using L-BFGS algorithm

6      $L\text{-}BFGS = \textbf{new } L\text{-}BFGSAlgorithm(f_r(\boldsymbol{x}), f_{\phi_k}(\boldsymbol{x}, \tilde{\boldsymbol{s}}_{\mathrm{mm}}), \tilde{\boldsymbol{s}}_{\mathrm{mm}}, \Omega)$ **repeat**
            // Perform one iteration of L-BFGS algorithm.
            // It calls Algorithm 4.2 for computation
            // of the objective function and the derivative

7         $L\text{-}BFGS.performIteration()$

8   **until** *Termination criterion*;

9      $\boldsymbol{s}_{\mathrm{mm}} = L\text{-}BFGS.getBestSolution()$

10 **end**

---

[2]http://vxl.sourceforge.net/

Algorithm 4.2: Objective function and derivative computation.

Input: $f_r(\boldsymbol{x}), f_{\phi_k}(\boldsymbol{x}, \tilde{\boldsymbol{s}}_{\mathrm{mm}}), \tilde{\boldsymbol{s}}_{\mathrm{mm}}, \Omega$

Output: $\mathcal{L}_{NCC}(\boldsymbol{s}_{\mathrm{mm}}), \frac{\partial \mathcal{L}_{NCC}(\boldsymbol{s}_{\mathrm{mm}})}{\partial \boldsymbol{s}_{\mathrm{mm}}}$

// Step 1: Computation of sum volume

1   $f(\boldsymbol{x}, \boldsymbol{s}_{\mathrm{mm}}) = \sum_{k=1}^{K} f_{\phi_k}(\boldsymbol{x}, \tilde{\boldsymbol{s}}_{\mathrm{mm}})$

// Step 2: Computation of objective function value

2 **foreach** $\boldsymbol{x} \in \Omega$ **do**

3     $n_{ff}(\boldsymbol{s}_{\mathrm{mm}}) = n_{ff}(\boldsymbol{s}_{\mathrm{mm}}) + f(\boldsymbol{x}, \boldsymbol{s}_{\mathrm{mm}})^2$

4     $n_{rr} \quad\;\; = n_{rr} + f_r(\boldsymbol{x})^2$

5     $n_{rf}(\boldsymbol{s}_{\mathrm{mm}}) = n_{rf}(\boldsymbol{s}_{\mathrm{mm}}) + f(\boldsymbol{x}, \boldsymbol{s}_{\mathrm{mm}}) \cdot f_r(\boldsymbol{x})$

6     $n_f(\boldsymbol{s}_{\mathrm{mm}}) = n_f(\boldsymbol{s}_{\mathrm{mm}}) + f(\boldsymbol{x}, \boldsymbol{s}_{\mathrm{mm}})$

7     $n_r \quad\;\; = n_r + f_r(\boldsymbol{x})$

8 **end**

9   $n_{ff}(\boldsymbol{s}_{\mathrm{mm}}) = n_{ff}(\boldsymbol{s}_{\mathrm{mm}}) + \frac{n_f(\boldsymbol{s}_{\mathrm{mm}})^2}{|\Omega|}$

10 $n_{rr} \quad\;\; = n_{rr} + \frac{n_r^2}{|\Omega|}$

11 $n_{rf}(\boldsymbol{s}_{\mathrm{mm}}) = n_{rf}(\boldsymbol{s}_{\mathrm{mm}}) + \frac{n_r \cdot n_f(\boldsymbol{s}_{\mathrm{mm}})}{|\Omega|}$

// Computation of objective function according to Equation 4.16

12 $\mathcal{L}_{NCC}(\boldsymbol{s}_{\mathrm{mm}}) = -\frac{n_{rf}(\boldsymbol{s}_{\mathrm{mm}})}{\sqrt{n_{rr} \cdot n_{ff}(\boldsymbol{s}_{\mathrm{mm}})}}$

// Step 3: Computation of derivative contribution

13 **foreach** $\boldsymbol{x} \in \Omega$ **do**

14   Compute $\kappa(\boldsymbol{x}, \boldsymbol{s}_{\mathrm{mm}})$ // according to Equation 4.26

15   Compute derivative $\frac{\partial \mathcal{L}_{NCC}(\boldsymbol{s}_{\mathrm{mm}})}{\partial \boldsymbol{s}_{\mathrm{mm},\boldsymbol{x}}}$ // according to Equation 4.25

16 **end**

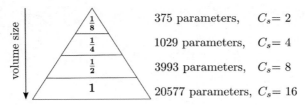

Figure 4.11: Registration pyramid for B-spline registration.

4.5.2.3   D-CR Parameter Setting

For the deformable B-Spline registration, a multi-resolution scheme of 4 levels is used with a sampling factor of 2 on each pyramid level. At the highest image resolution a number of $C_s = 16$ control points are used in each spatial dimension. The choice of C_s highly influences the relation of smoothness (small C_s) to flexibility (large C_s) of the motion. The imaging pyramid and the resulting number of parameters as well as the resulting spatial resolution is shown in Figure 4.11.

Here, a toolbox called `elastix`[3] for non-rigid registration of medical images is used for the 3-D/3-D motion estimation [Klei 10]. The adaptive stochastic gradient descent optimizer is set to a certain number of iterations, empirical experiments showed that $W = 500$ iterations on each pyramid level are sufficient to result in a minimal objective function value. For the remaining parameters, the default settings were used.

The motion vector field was only estimated inside a region of interest (ROI) where the heart motion is expected, therefore, a regional mask Ω is defined. In this first implementation the mask volume is generated manually by the user.

4.6   Evaluation and Results

In the following sections, the evaluation of the different motion estimation algorithms with respect to the reconstruction quality is presented.

4.6.1   Datasets

Two different kinds of datasets were used for motion estimation and compensation evaluation, simulated phantom datasets, and clinical porcine models. A first clinical patient dataset is discussed non-competitively in Section 4.7.

4.6.1.1   Ventricular Phantoms

Several different phantom datasets were created, and a short overview is given in Table 4.3. In general, ventricle datasets [Mlle 13b, Maie 12, Maie 13] of a similar design to the XCAT phantom [Sega 08] are simulated. The phantom is defined by cubic B-splines, as well as the cardiac motion. The cardiac motion is extracted from

---

[3]http://elastix.isi.uu.nl/about.php

Dataset	Description of the phantom dataset
d_1	Dynamic monochromatic without catheter (with noise)
$d_{1,GT}$	Static monochromatic without catheter for each heart phase (no noise)
d_2	Dynamic polychromatic with catheter (with noise)
$d_{2,GT}$	Static polychromatic phantom catheter for each heart phase (no noise)

Table 4.3: Overview of the different generated phantom datasets.

the XCAT phantom. For the first phantom dataset d_1, it is assumed that all materials have the same spectral absorption behavior as water. The density of the contrasted left ventricle bloodpool was set to $2.5\,g/cm^3$, the density of the myocardial wall to $1.5\,g/cm^3$ and the contrasted blood in the aorta to $2.0\,g/cm^3$. Data was simulated using a clinical protocol with the following parameters: the acquisition time was 14.5 s capturing 381 projection images with an angular increment of 0.52° during one C-arm rotation [De B 13b]. The isotropic pixel resolution was 0.31 mm/pixel (0.19 mm in isocenter) and the detector size 1240 × 960 pixel. The heart rate was simulated with 131 bpm. A total of 32 heart cycles were acquired resulting in a number of reconstructed heart phases $K = 12$. Image reconstruction was performed on an image volume of $(25.6\ cm)^3$ distributed on a 256^3 voxel grid.

Additionally, a phantom dataset is simulated with a polychromatic X-ray spectrum. A source spectrum $E(b)$ with $b \in [1,\ 36]$ from 10 keV to 90 keV, and a time current product of 2.5 mAs per X-ray pulse are used. The material of the anode disk is assumed to be tungsten and the half value layer thickness was measured to fit to a clinical C-arm system (Axiom Artis dTA C-arm system, Siemens AG, Healthcare Sector, Forchheim, Germany). A catheter is simulated coming from the aorta into the left ventricle. The same deformation field as for the heart was applied to the catheter. The material of the catheter is similar to copper in order to induce severe streak artifacts in the reconstructions. The catheter, bones and the bone marrow, have the material properties according to the mass attenuation coefficients of the NIST X-Ray Table[4]. For all other structures it is assumed that they have the same absorption behavior as water with different densities similar to the FORBILD phantom[5]. The density of the ventricular bloodpool, myocardium and aorta is the same as in the monochromatic simulations. The same imaging protocol as for the monochromatic phantom data was used for simulation.

Poisson distributed noise was added to the simulated projection stacks such that the noise characteristics of the reconstructed images fit those of the clinical data. As gold standard, static projection images were generated without noise. The phantom projection data and geometry are publicly available[6].

An example of the generated phantom in 3-D image space is shown in Figures 4.12a and 4.12b. Two example projection images of the simulated phantom without the catheter and with the catheter are shown in Figures 4.12c and 4.12d.

---

[4]http://physics.nist.gov/PhysRefData/Xcom/html/xcom1.html
[5]http://www.imp.uni-erlangen.de/phantoms/thorax/thorax.htm
[6]http://conrad.stanford.edu/data/heart

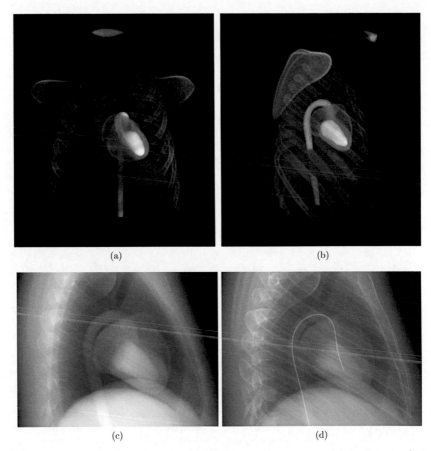

Figure 4.12: Example images of the simulated phantom datasets. (a) Anterior view of the generated monochromatic phantom dataset. (b) Left sagittal view of the generated phantom dataset with the catheter. (c) Simulated 2-D projection image, with contrasted LV, myocardium and aorta and (d) simulated 2-D projection image of catheter phantom.

4.6.1.2 Porcine Models

The methods were also applied to two experimental datasets of porcine models (p_1, p_2). Image acquisition was performed using an Artis zee system (Siemens AG, Healthcare Sector, Forchheim, Germany) at a research laboratory at the University of Leuven, Belgium. The acquisition time was 14.5 s capturing 381 projection images with 30 f/s, and an angular increment of 0.52° during one C-arm sweep [De B 13b]. The isotropic pixel resolution was 0.31 mm/pixel (0.19 mm in isocenter) and the detector size 1240 × 960 pixel. The heart rate was stimulated through external heart pacing to 131 bpm. A total of 32 heart cycles were acquired resulting in a number of reconstructed heart phases of $K = 12$. A total volume of about 150 ml contrast agent fluid was administered intravenously at a speed of 10 ml/s (p_1) and 7 ml/s (p_2), respectively, 5 s (p_1) and 10 s (p_2) before the X-ray rotation was started. The total contrast injection time was 15 s (p_1) and 21 s (p_2). Image reconstruction was performed on an image volume of $(25.6 \text{ cm})^3$ distributed on a 256^3 voxel grid.

4.6.2 Quantitative Evaluation Methods of 3-D Reconstruction Quality

For the dynamic phantom data, the 3-D normalized (nRMSE) and the relative root mean square error (rRMSE) and the 3-D universal image quality index (UQI) were evaluated. In order to measure only the artifacts introduced by the heart motion, the non-gated and noise-free FDK reconstruction using all projections of the static heart phantom of the same heart phase is used as gold standard. The nRMSE, the rRMSE as well as the UQI were evaluated inside a manually selected region of interest (ROI) denoted as Ω around the ventricle. For the phantom with the catheter, a static phantom of the different heart phases was created without the catheter and used as gold standard. The region of the catheter is also excluded from the evaluation, in order to focus on motion artifacts at the heart walls. The quality of the removal of the catheter if performed is not the focus of this study. Let $f_{\text{GS},\phi_k}(\boldsymbol{x})$ be the function which returns the intensity value of the gold standard image for a certain heart phase and $f_T(\boldsymbol{x}, \boldsymbol{s})$ the function to be evaluated.

4.6.2.1 Normalized Root Mean Square Error (nRMSE)

The normalized root mean square error (nRMSE) was used to quantify the 3-D reconstruction error of the motion-compensated reconstructions or standard FDK reconstructions compared to the gold standard FDK of the static phantom. The nRMSE can be computed as follows

$$\text{nRMSE}_{\phi_k} = \zeta \cdot \sqrt{\frac{1}{|\Omega|} \sum_{x \in \Omega} \left(f_{\text{GS},\phi_k}(\boldsymbol{x}) - f_T(\boldsymbol{x}, \boldsymbol{s}) \right)^2}, \text{ with} \qquad (4.40)$$

$$\zeta = \frac{1}{\max_{x \in \Omega} \left(f_{\text{GS},\phi_k}(\boldsymbol{x}) \right) - \min_{x \in \Omega} \left(f_{\text{GS},\phi_k}(\boldsymbol{x}) \right)}, \qquad (4.41)$$

where $|\Omega|$ denotes the number of voxels inside the region of interest (ROI). All results were averaged over the heart phases, resulting in the overall nRMSE.

4.6.2.2 Relative Root Mean Square Error (rRMSE)

The relative root mean square error (rRMSE) was used to quantify the 3-D reconstruction error as

$$\text{rRMSE}_{\phi_k} = \sqrt{\frac{1}{|\Omega|} \sum_{x \in \Omega} \left(\frac{f_{\text{GS},\phi_k}(\boldsymbol{x}) - f_T(\boldsymbol{x}, \boldsymbol{s})}{f_{\text{GS},\phi_k}(\boldsymbol{x})} \right)^2}, \tag{4.42}$$

where $|\Omega|$ denotes the number of voxels inside the ROI. For an overall rRMSE, all results were averaged over the heart phases ϕ_k.

4.6.2.3 Universal Quality Index (UQI)

As a 3-D image quality metric the universal image quality index (UQI) was computed [Wang 02]. The UQI ranges from -1 to 1, where 1 is the best value achieved when $f_{\text{GS},\phi_k}(\boldsymbol{x}) = f_T(\boldsymbol{x}, \boldsymbol{s})$ for all $\boldsymbol{x}$ inside the defined ROI. The UQI is defined as

$$\text{UQI}_{\phi_k} = \frac{4 \cdot \sigma_{ff_{\text{GS}}} \cdot \overline{f}_T \cdot \overline{f}_{\text{GS}}}{\left(\sigma_f^2 + \sigma_{f_{\text{GS}}}^2 \right) \left[(\overline{f}_T)^2 + (\overline{f}_{\text{GS}})^2 \right]}, \tag{4.43}$$

where $\overline{f}_T$, $\overline{f}_{\text{GS}}$ represent the mean values, σ_f^2, $\sigma_{f_{\text{GS}}}^2$ the variances, and $\sigma_{ff_{\text{GS}}}$ the cross correlation inside the ROI. For an overall UQI, all results were averaged over the heart phases ϕ_k.

4.6.3 Edge Response Function

For the datasets, the edge response functions are evaluated, since the motion-compensated reconstructions improve the sharpness of the edges.

4.6.3.1 Definition for Phantom Data

Mean Edge Sharpness Δ. For analysis of edge profiles the start and end points $x_{i,1}$ and $x_{i,2}$ at the lateral wall of the ventricle are determined in the gold standard reconstruction and used for all other images. Here, a number of lines were taken orthogonal to the lateral wall. The slope $m_{i,\text{GS}}$ is computed between these two points

$$m_{i,\text{GS}} = \frac{\Delta y_i}{\Delta x_i} = \frac{y_{i,2} - y_{i,1}}{x_{i,2} - x_{i,1}}. \tag{4.44}$$

For the motion-compensated reconstructions, also the slope m_i between the two points $x_{i,1}$, $x_{i,2}$ is determined. Consequently, the deviation Δ_i between the slopes m_i and the $m_{i,\text{GS}}$ can be computed by

$$\Delta_i = \frac{|m_{i,\text{GS}} - m_i|}{|m_{i,\text{GS}}|}, \tag{4.45}$$

$$\Delta = \frac{1}{L} \sum_{i=1}^{L} \Delta_i, \tag{4.46}$$

where L denotes the number of lines. In order to stabilize the result, and to eliminate small outliers, several lines are taken and the deviation Δ_i is measured individually for each line. Afterwards, the edge sharpness deviation Δ_i for each line is averaged to determine the mean edge sharpness deviation Δ. Furthermore, in order to exclude outliers, the median of Δ_i is also quoted as Q_Δ.

Mean edge error τ. For the phantom data it is also possible to measure the accuracy and trend of the edge between each motion-compensated reconstruction and the gold standard. This is done by appropriately modifying Equation (4.42), here the gold standard edge value is denoted as $y_{\text{GT},j}$ and the edge profile to be tested y_j

$$\tau_i = \sqrt{\frac{1}{\Delta x_i} \sum_{j=x_{i,1}}^{x_{i,2}} \left(\frac{y_{\text{GT},j} - y_j}{y_{\text{GT},j}}\right)^2} \tag{4.47}$$

$$\tau = \frac{1}{L} \sum_{i=1}^{L} \tau_i. \tag{4.48}$$

The mean error τ of the trend of the edge profile and the median (Q_τ) are computed.

4.6.3.2   Definition for Porcine Data

Mean Edge Sharpness Λ. For the analysis of the edge response profile of the porcine models a similar sharpness measure as for the phantom is used. However, no gold standard edge is known. Therefore, again a line profile is computed along a reference line i for each motion-compensated reconstruction. Each line is filtered with a Gaussian kernel in order to remove small outliers. In the filtered line profile the beginning $x_{i,1}$ and the end $x_{i,2}$ of the edge are determined, as minimum and maximum points. The resulting slope m_i between these two points $x_{i,1}$, $x_{i,2}$ is computed, but the values from the non-filtered line are used. In order to stabilize the result, and to eliminate small outliers, several lines are taken and the m_i is measured individually for each line. Afterwards, the edge sharpness m_i for each line is averaged to determine the mean edge sharpness, denoted with Λ

$$m_i = \frac{\Delta y_i}{\Delta x_i} = \frac{y_{i,2} - y_{i,1}}{x_{i,2} - x_{i,1}}, \tag{4.49}$$

$$\Lambda = \frac{1}{L} \sum_{i=1}^{L} m_i. \tag{4.50}$$

Furthermore, in order to exclude outliers, the median Q_Λ is also provided.

4.6.4   Experimental Results

In this section, the quantitative and qualitative results for the two phantom datasets and the two porcine models are presented.

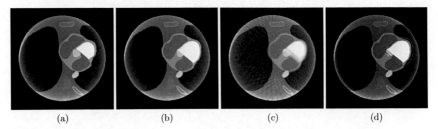

(a)	(b)	(c)	(d)

Figure 4.13: Central slice of (a) the non-gated FDK result of static phantom 30 % without noise (b) the non-gated FDK result of static phantom 80 % without noise, (c) the non-gated FDK result of the dynamic phantom reconstruction of the phantom model without a catheter and with noise and (d) an example of the used ROI (W 3100 HU, C 780 HU, slice thickness 1 mm).

4.6.4.1 Phantom Data without Catheter

Visual Inspection. The gold standard reconstruction of the phantom data without the catheter at a heart phase of 30 % and of 80 % are illustrated in Figure 4.13a and 4.13b. The non-gated FDK reconstruction has motion blur around the left ventricle and the myocardial wall is hardly visible in Figure 4.13c. An example of the defined regin of interest for the quantitative evaluation is given in Figure 4.13d. The initial images and the motion-compensated results are presented in Figure 4.14. In Figure 4.14c, the gated FDK depicts the myocardial wall, but is severely degraded by noise and streak artifacts. The FFDK and FV have less streak artifact and a lower noise level, but have a smoother image impression compared to the non-gated FDK reconstruction, cf. Figures 4.14e and 4.14g. Motion compensation almost eliminates streak artifacts and further reduces the noise level, see Figures 4.14d, 4.14f and 4.14h. The CR-CMC reconstruction result at heart phase 30 % is given in Figure 4.14a. The reconstruction shows a good delineation of the left ventricle. In Figure 4.14b, the results for the CMHPR-MC are presented. The reconstruction shows a sharper outline of the ventricular border and has a smoother appearance compared to the non-gated FDK. This can be due to the used reference image, the FV reconstruction in Figure 4.14g also has a smoother appearance compared to the non-gated FDK reconstruction. The CR-CMC and the D-CR reconstructions with different initial images (FDK-MC, FFDK-MC and FV-MC) show comparable and good delineation of the left ventricle, cf. Figures 4.14a, 4.14d, 4.14f, and 4.14h. Almost no difference can be seen for the D-CR when using different initial images.

The same observations can be made for the phantom data at a relative heart phase of 80% in Figures 4.14i to 4.14p.

Quantitative Results. The results of the monochromatic phantom without a catheter are given in Table 4.4. The CMHPR and CMHPR-MC reconstruction show minor improvement compared to the non-gated FDK volumes. The FDK reconstruction highly suffers from noise and streak artifacts, visible in a high rRMSE and lower UQI value. The CR-CMC, the FFDK-MC and the FV-MC reconstructions achieve

Method	nRMSE	rRMSE	UQI
CR-CMC	**0.042 ± 0.01**	**0.08 ± 0.01**	**0.98 ± 0.01**
CMHPR	0.056 ± 0.01	0.10 ± 0.01	0.97 ± 0.01
CMHPR-MC	0.055 ± 0.01	0.10 ± 0.01	0.97 ± 0.01
FDK-MC	0.046 ± 0.01	0.09 ± 0.02	**0.98 ± 0.01**
FFDK-MC	0.046 ± 0.01	**0.08 ± 0.02**	**0.98 ± 0.01**
FV-MC	0.046 ± 0.01	**0.08 ± 0.02**	**0.98 ± 0.01**
FDK	0.075 ± 0.01	0.14 ± 0.01	0.95 ± 0.01
FFDK	0.059 ± 0.01	0.10 ± 0.02	0.97 ± 0.01
FV	0.057 ±0.01	0.10 ± 0.01	0.97 ± 0.01
non-gated FDK	0.063 ± 0.01	0.12 ± 0.04	0.96 ± 0.01

Table 4.4: The rRMSE and UQI of the dynamic phantom model without a catheter for all $K = 12$ heart phases as mean and standard deviation. The best values are marked in bold.

comparable good results, and the image quality improved with respect to the initial images. The FDK-MC has a slightly inferior rRMSE value, but the same nRMSE and UQI result as the FFDK-MC and FV-MC.

In Table 4.5, the mean edge sharpness deviation Δ is given for the phantom data without a catheter. For the systolic heart phase, the FDK-MC, the FFDK-MC, and the FV-MC achieve the best result. The result of the mean edge sharpness of the FDK and the FFDK highly depend on the distribution of the streaks, if a streak crosses exactly at the edge of the profile, the sharpness measure is deteriorated. The FV initial volume results vary between both heart phases and hence provides no stable results. The CR-CMC result also varies slightly between both heart phases, and shows a slightly increased deviation compared to the FDK-MC. The CMHPR and the motion-compensated reconstruction (CMHPR-MC) improve the sharpness of the endocardium compared to the non-gated FDK reconstruction, however, results in higher sharpness deviations, especially in the systolic heart phase. The mean error τ of the edge profiles is given in Table 4.6. The best results are achieved with the FDK-MC, FFDK-MC and FV-MC reconstructions. The FDK and FFDK edge profiles are highly corrupted by noise and show a higher deviation compared to the gold standard edge profile. It can be seen that the CMHPR and CMHPR-MC reconstructions have the same or even a smaller deviation compared to the gold standard than the initial volumes. The FDK-MC, FFDK-MC and the FV-MC achieve slightly inferior results than the CR-CMC reconstructions.

4.6.4.2   Phantom Data with Catheter

Visual Inspection. For the phantom dataset with the simulated catheter the results are shown in Figure 4.15 for a relative heart phase of 30 %. The gold standard

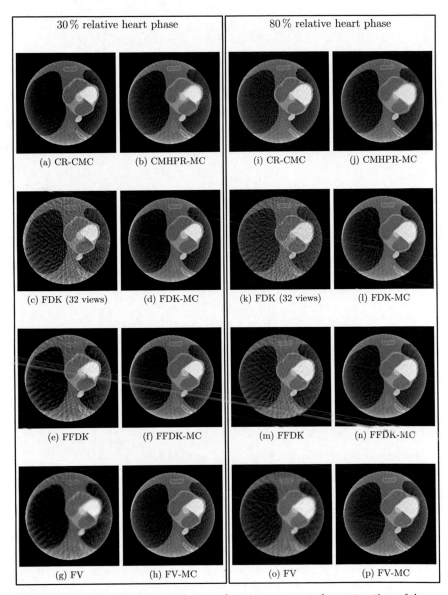

Figure 4.14: Central slice of initial volumes and motion-compensated reconstructions of the phantom model without any catheter at a relative heart phase of about 30 % and 80 % (W 3100 HU, C 780 HU, slice thickness 1 mm).

Method	Δ_{ϕ_3}	$Q_{\Delta_{\phi_3}}$	Δ_{ϕ_9}	$Q_{\Delta_{\phi_9}}$
CR-CMC	0.16 ± 0.13	0.10	0.06 ± 0.06	0.04
CMHPR	0.25 ± 0.05	0.23	0.11 ± 0.03	0.10
CMHPR-MC	0.20 ± 0.06	0.18	0.10 ± 0.03	0.10
FDK-MC	$\mathbf{0.09 \pm 0.10}$	$\mathbf{0.06}$	$\mathbf{0.05 \pm 0.05}$	$\mathbf{0.03}$
FFDK-MC	0.10 ± 0.07	0.09	$\mathbf{0.05 \pm 0.05}$	0.04
FV-MC	0.15 ± 0.13	0.10	$\mathbf{0.05 \pm 0.04}$	0.04
FDK	0.18 ± 0.12	0.17	0.18 ± 0.05	0.17
FFDK	0.30 ± 0.07	0.30	0.08 ± 0.08	0.05
FV	0.16 ± 0.09	0.14	$\mathbf{0.02 \pm 0.02}$	$\mathbf{0.02}$
non-gated FDK	0.65 ± 0.05	0.65	0.32 ± 0.10	0.32

Table 4.5: The mean (Δ) and the median (Q_Δ) edge sharpness deviation of the dynamic phantom model without a catheter compared to the gold standard at heart phases $\phi_3 \approx 30\,\%$ and $\phi_9 \approx 80\,\%$. The best values are marked in bold.

Method	τ_{ϕ_3}	$Q_{\tau_{\phi_3}}$	τ_{ϕ_9}	$Q_{\tau_{\phi_9}}$
CR-CMC	0.13 ± 0.03	0.12	0.07 ± 0.02	0.07
CMHPR	0.14 ± 0.05	0.14	0.08 ± 0.01	0.08
CMHPR-MC	0.14 ± 0.05	0.13	0.07 ± 0.01	0.08
FDK-MC	$\mathbf{0.09 \pm 0.02}$	$\mathbf{0.08}$	0.07 ± 0.02	0.07
FFDK-MC	$\mathbf{0.09 \pm 0.03}$	$\mathbf{0.08}$	0.07 ± 0.02	0.07
FV-MC	0.12 ± 0.04	0.10	$\mathbf{0.06 \pm 0.02}$	$\mathbf{0.06}$
FDK	0.19 ± 0.06	0.20	0.34 ± 0.08	0.34
FFDK	0.18 ± 0.03	0.18	0.30 ± 0.09	0.33
FV	0.14 ± 0.04	0.13	0.19 ± 0.04	0.18
non-gated FDK	0.54 ± 0.11	0.56	0.19 ± 0.03	0.19

Table 4.6: The mean error (τ) and the median (Q_τ) of the accuracy of the dynamic phantom model without a catheter of the edge profile compared to the gold standard at heart phases $\phi_3 \approx 30\,\%$ and $\phi_9 \approx 80\,\%$. The best values are marked in bold.

reconstruction is given in Figure 4.15a. The non-gated FDK volume suffers from the motion artifacts around the left ventricle, cf. Figure 4.15b. The catheter causes severe streak artifacts in the non-filtered and filtered ECG-gated reconstructions, see Figures 4.15e and 4.15i. Some initial images are less sensitive to the catheter. The FV, cathFDK and cathFFDK in Figures 4.15g, 4.15k and 4.15m show less streak artifact. Consequently, the corresponding motion compensated images show a much better image quality than the results of the FDK-MC and FFDK-MC reconstruction, see Figures 4.15h, 4.15l and 4.15n. In Figures 4.15f and 4.15j can be seen that the FDK-MC and FFDK-MC reconstructions suffer from streak artifacts induced by the catheter and motion compensation does not eliminate these streak artifacts since the motion estimation is disturbed by them, cf. Figures 4.15f and 4.15j. Overall, the cathFDK-MC, cathFFDK-MC and FV-MC show comparably good results. In Figure 4.15c, the CR-CMC results shows a sharp ventricular boundary, but still has minor streak artifacts. The result of the CMHPR-MC in Figure 4.15d has a smoother visual appearance compared to the non-gated FDK of the dynamic phantom and is more similar to the FV volume in Figure 4.15g, which is used as reference volume.

Quantitative Results.   For the phantom dataset with the simulated catheter, the results of the nRMSE, rRMSE and the UQI are given in Table 4.7. For brevity, in the table only the quality values between the different motion-compensated reconstructions are illustrated. The FDK-MC and the FFDK-MC have a higher rRMSE value compared to the other motion-compensated reconstructions, due to the fact that some streak artifacts are registered onto each other and result in streak artifacts in the final motion-compensated reconstruction. The same can be seen for the UQI values. The smallest nRMSE, but highest rRMSE value was achieved by the CMHPR-MC. A slightly inferior nRMSE and the smallest rRMSE was achieved by the cathFDK-MC. Only slightly inferior results are given by the cathFFDK-MC and the FV-MC. The CR-CMC reconstructions achieve a small rRMSE value and a high UQI value, however, the rRMSE value is higher than the FV-MC, cathFDK-MC, and cathFFDK-MC reconstructions. The CMHPR-MC has less streak artifacts compared to the FDK-MC and the FFDK-MC, but results in a higher error compared to the cathFDK-MC, cathFFDK-MC and FV-MC. The UQI values vary only slightly among the motion-compensated reconstructions except for the FDK-MC and the FFDK-MC.

Table 4.8 shows the results for the mean edge sharpness deviation Δ measurements of the phantom with the catheter. The reference lines and the mean edge profile are given in Figure 4.16. The best result is given by the FV-MC approach and the cathFDK-MC. The CR-CMC still shows minor streak artifacts at the lateral wall and achieves minor sharpness values. It is again visible that the FDK-MC and the FFDK-MC approach have slightly divergent sharpness compared to the gold standard due to the streak artifacts inside the reconstructions. These artifacts cause outliers in the line profiles and a higher standard deviation in the sharpness measurements. The cathFFDK-MC shows no improvement compared to the non-filtered version of cathFDK-MC, which may be due to smoothing out of small structure of the myocardium in the initial images which cannot be recovered in the motion-compensated reconstruction. The CMHPR-MC has slightly inferior edge sharpness

Method	nRMSE	rRMSE	UQI
CR-CMC	0.103 ± 0.01	0.67 ± 0.55	$\mathbf{0.94 \pm 0.01}$
CMHPR-MC	$\mathbf{0.096 \pm 0.01}$	0.74 ± 0.60	$\mathbf{0.94 \pm 0.01}$
FDK-MC	0.174 ± 0.01	0.85 ± 0.34	0.84 ± 0.01
FFDK-MC	0.157 ± 0.01	0.84 ± 0.33	0.87 ± 0.01
FV-MC	0.112 ± 0.01	0.63 ± 0.28	0.93 ± 0.01
cathFDK-MC	0.107 ± 0.01	$\mathbf{0.62 \pm 0.43}$	$\mathbf{0.94 \pm 0.01}$
cathFFDK-MC	0.108 ± 0.01	0.63 ± 0.37	0.93 ± 0.01

Table 4.7: The rRMSE and UQI of the dynamic phantom model with a catheter for all $K = 12$ heart phases as mean and standard deviation. The best values are marked in bold.

results compared to the cathFDK-MC result and varies in sharpness between the two heart phases.

In Table 4.9, the mean error τ of the edge profiles between the phantom reconstructions and the gold standard reconstructions is given. The CMHPR-MC has the same mean error τ as the cathFDK-MC result, however, it varies between the two heart phases. The best result was again performed with the cathFDK-MC. The remaining streak artifacts slightly hamper the CR-CMC reconstruction. The FV-MC and the cathFFDK-MC result in slightly inferior results as compared to the cathFDK-MC.

Overall, the cathFDK-MC, cathFFDK-MC and the FV-MC differ only slightly when considering all quantitative results. The CR-CMC achieves slightly inferior results compared to the cathFDK-MC, cathFFDK-MC and the FV-MC. Given the results for the CMHPR-MC, the error is inferior compared to the cathFDK-MC, the cathFFDK-MC, the FV-MC, and the CR-CMC. The FDK-MC and FFDK-MC are slightly degraded by streak artifacts which are still present after the motion-compensated reconstruction.

4.6.4.3   Porcine Data

Visual Inspection. The non-gated FDK reconstruction of the porcine data p_1 illustrates a doubled catheter and blurred endocardium edges, since the non-gated FDK reconstruction averages over all heart phases, cf. Figure 4.17a. The motion-compensated reconstruction of the CR-CMC algorithm is shown in Figure 4.17b. In Figure 4.17c, the result of the CMHPR-MC is given. The visual appearance of the endocardial boundary is smoother than in the other motion-compensated reconstructions. An improvement is achieved compared to the initial gated FDK reconstructions. The gated FDK displays the sharp contours of the endocardium, however, prominent streak artifacts are apparent, cf. Figure 4.17d. A better result is provided by the FFDK and FV reconstruction in Figure 4.17h and 4.17f. However, both exhibit blurred streak artifacts and are severely smoothed. Looking at the cathFDK reconstruction in Figure 4.17j, the artifacts from the catheter are removed, but the noise is still present in the volume. The noise is reduced in the cathFFDK volume

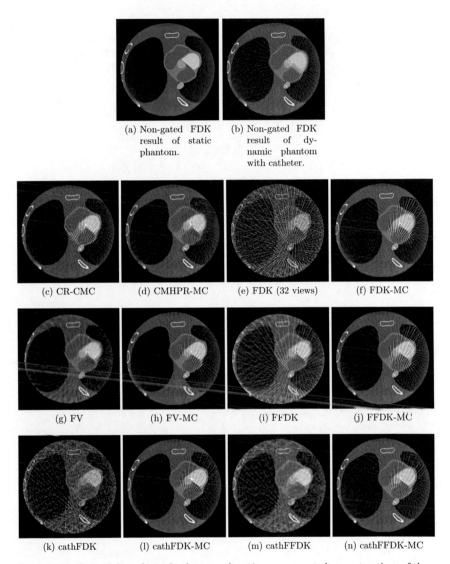

Figure 4.15: Central slice of initial volumes and motion-compensated reconstructions of the phantom model with a catheter at a relative heart phase of about 30 % (W 3100 HU, C 780 HU, slice thickness 1 mm).

Method	Δ_{ϕ_3}	$Q_{\Delta_{\phi_3}}$	Δ_{ϕ_9}	$Q_{\Delta_{\phi_9}}$
CR-CMC	0.21 ± 0.12	0.18	0.21 ± 0.18	0.21
CMHPR-MC	0.12 ± 0.06	0.13	0.22 ± 0.15	0.19
FDK-MC	0.20 ± 0.12	0.19	0.34 ± 0.16	0.32
FFDK-MC	0.14 ± 0.10	0.15	0.18 ± 0.14	0.21
FV-MC	$\mathbf{0.11 \pm 0.07}$	$\mathbf{0.07}$	0.11 ± 0.07	0.10
cathFDK-MC	0.14 ± 0.05	0.16	$\mathbf{0.07 \pm 0.05}$	$\mathbf{0.07}$
cathFFDK-MC	0.15 ± 0.13	0.11	0.09 ± 0.06	0.09

Table 4.8: The mean (Δ) and the median (Q_Δ) edge sharpness deviation of the dynamic phantom model with a catheter compared to the gold standard at heart phases $\phi_3 \approx 30\,\%$ and $\phi_9 \approx 80\,\%$. The best values are marked in bold.

Method	τ_{ϕ_3}	$Q_{\tau_{\phi_3}}$	τ_{ϕ_9}	$Q_{\tau_{\phi_9}}$
CR-CMC	0.42 ± 0.25	0.36	0.29 ± 0.04	0.30
CMHPR-MC	$\mathbf{0.26 \pm 0.10}$	0.26	0.33 ± 0.07	0.31
FDK-MC	0.47 ± 0.20	0.44	0.59 ± 0.18	0.63
FFDK-MC	0.39 ± 0.13	0.38	0.48 ± 0.14	0.52
FV-MC	0.28 ± 0.15	$\mathbf{0.21}$	0.28 ± 0.06	0.28
cathFDK-MC	$\mathbf{0.26 \pm 0.15}$	0.25	$\mathbf{0.25 \pm 0.04}$	$\mathbf{0.24}$
cathFFDK-MC	0.27 ± 0.17	0.26	0.28 ± 0.10	0.28

Table 4.9: The mean error (τ) and the median (Q_τ) of the accuracy of the dynamic phantom model with a catheter of the edge profile compared to the gold standard at heart phases $\phi_3 \approx 30\,\%$ and $\phi_9 \approx 80\,\%$. The best values are marked in bold.

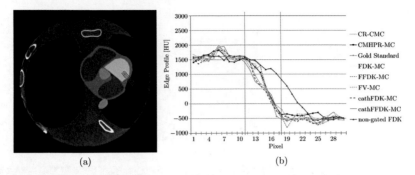

(a)   (b)

Figure 4.16: Measurements of the edge response profile for the catheter phantom. (a) Visualized lines for edge response function and sharpness for the catheter phantom. (b) Mean edge response profile for phantom dataset with catheter of the different motion compensation algorithms at 30 % heart phase.

in Figure 4.17l. The motion-compensated reconstructions yield improved results, cf. Figures 4.17e, 4.17g, 4.17i, 4.17k and 4.17m. Overall, there is not much difference in image quality for the CR-CMC, the FV-MC, the cathFDK-MC and the cathFFDK-MC, only the intensities of the remaining streak artifacts vary slightly. The same can be seen for the reconstruction of p_1 at a heart phase of 80 % in Figure 4.18 and the second porcine model p_2 at a heart phase of 20 % in Figure 4.19 and at a heart phase of 80 % in Figure 4.20.

Since it is now possible to reconstruct a varying number of heart phases with improved image quality, the dynamics of the heart can be visualized and analyzed. Different heart phase reconstructions of the porcine model p_1 with the cathFDK-MC are given in Figure 4.21.

Quantitative Results.   In Table 4.10, the results for the sharpness measures are given for the clinical data. An example of the reference lines and the resulting mean edge profile is illustrated in Figure 4.22. The cathFFDK-MC and the CR-CMC have the steepest edge, however the cathFDK-MC also has a well delineated edge profile and differs only slightly. The CR-CMC edge sharpness for p_1 is inferior compared to the cathFDK-MC approach, however, CR-CMC shows a high standard deviation compared to the cathFDK-MC approach for p_2. The FDK-MC and the FFDK-MC images result in slightly inferior results for both datasets due to the different magnitude of streaking artifacts, e.g., a catheter or a pacing electrode. The FV-MC exhibits a high variation between the two porcine models and hence produces no stable results. The CMHPR-MC provides no reliable edge information, cf. Figure 4.22b. This might be due to the fact that the reference image (FV) already misses this information and, thus, the CMHPR-MC cannot recover it.

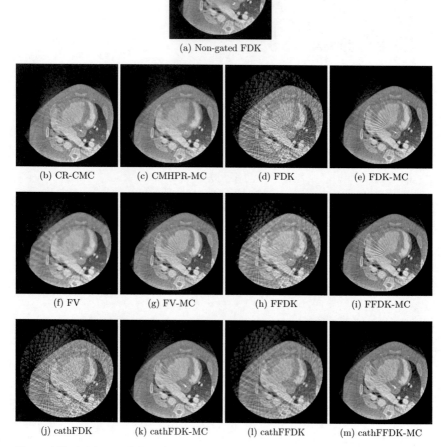

(a) Non-gated FDK

(b) CR-CMC   (c) CMHPR-MC   (d) FDK   (e) FDK-MC

(f) FV   (g) FV-MC   (h) FFDK   (i) FFDK-MC

(j) cathFDK   (k) cathFDK-MC   (l) cathFFDK   (m) cathFFDK-MC

Figure 4.17: Axial central slice of initial volumes and motion-compensated reconstructions of porcine model p_1 at a relative heart phase of about 30% (W 2400 HU, C 226 HU, slice thickness 1 mm). The image data was provided by Prof. Dr. Heidbüchel and Dr. De Buck from the University of Leuven, Belgium.

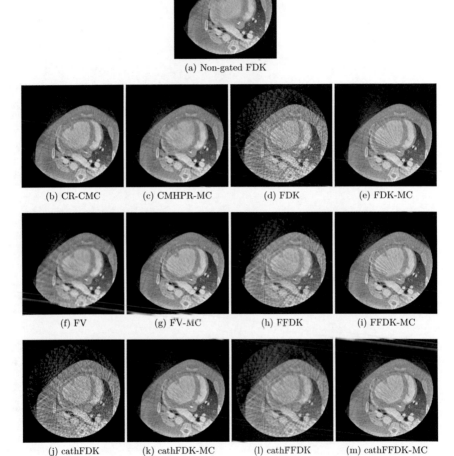

(a) Non-gated FDK

(b) CR-CMC   (c) CMHPR-MC   (d) FDK   (e) FDK-MC

(f) FV   (g) FV-MC   (h) FFDK   (i) FFDK-MC

(j) cathFDK   (k) cathFDK-MC   (l) cathFFDK   (m) cathFFDK-MC

Figure 4.18: Axial central slice of initial volumes and motion-compensated reconstructions of porcine model p_1 at a relative heart phase of about 80% (W 2400 HU, C 226 HU, slice thickness 1 mm). The image data was provided by Prof. Dr. Heidbüchel and Dr. De Buck from the University of Leuven, Belgium.

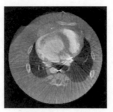

(a) Non-gated FDK

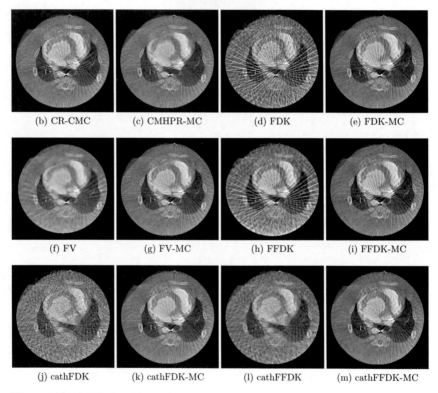

(b) CR-CMC   (c) CMHPR-MC   (d) FDK   (e) FDK-MC

(f) FV   (g) FV-MC   (h) FFDK   (i) FFDK-MC

(j) cathFDK   (k) cathFDK-MC   (l) cathFFDK   (m) cathFFDK-MC

Figure 4.19: Axial slice 28 mm from the central slice of initial volumes and motion-compensated reconstructions of porcine model p_2 at a relative heart phase of about 20 % (W 2400 HU, C 226 HU, slice thickness 1 mm). The image data was provided by Prof. Dr. Heidbüchel and Dr. De Buck from the University of Leuven, Belgium.

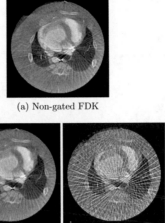

(a) Non-gated FDK

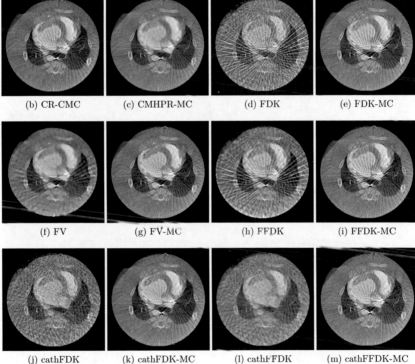

(b) CR-CMC   (c) CMHPR-MC   (d) FDK   (e) FDK-MC

(f) FV   (g) FV-MC   (h) FFDK   (i) FFDK-MC

(j) cathFDK   (k) cathFDK-MC   (l) cathFFDK   (m) cathFFDK-MC

Figure 4.20: Axial slice 28 mm from the central slice of initial volumes and motion-compensated reconstructions of porcine model p_2 at a relative heart phase of about 80 % (W 2400 HU, C 226 HU, slice thickness 1 mm). The image data was provided by Prof. Dr. Heidbüchel and Dr. De Buck from the University of Leuven, Belgium.

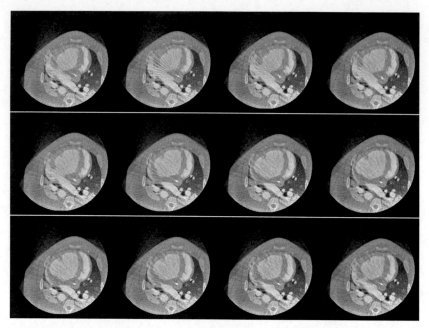

Figure 4.21: Illustration of different heart phases of porcine model p_1 reconstructed using the cathFDK-MC method (W 2400 HU, C 226 HU, slice thickness 1 mm). A number of $K = 12$ heart phases representing one heart cycle. Starting at a relative heart phase of about 10 % (left upper corner) and continuing from left to right and top to bottom with a relative heart phase increment of about $\frac{1}{12} \cdot 100$ %. The image data was provided by Prof. Dr. Heidbüchel and Dr. De Buck from the University of Leuven, Belgium.

	p_1		p_2	
Method	Λ_{ϕ_3}	$Q_{\Lambda_{\phi_3}}$	Λ_{ϕ_3}	$Q_{\Lambda_{\phi_9}}$
CR-CMC	24.81 ± 6.40	26.85	$\mathbf{52.22 \pm 10.42}$	**52.32**
CMHPR-MC	15.15 ± 4.96	14.54	12.06 ± 6.93	12.16
FDK-MC	24.18 ± 7.02	23.85	42.20 ± 9.42	42.64
FFDK-MC	24.33 ± 2.15	24.12	45.46 ± 11.9	39.52
FV-MC	22.44 ± 4.76	21.20	48.44 ± 4.58	47.73
cathFDK-MC	25.04 ± 8.21	27.57	47.82 ± 3.95	**48.52**
cathFFDK-MC	$\mathbf{26.60 \pm 7.26}$	**28.55**	49.45 ± 5.26	47.69

Table 4.10: The mean (Λ) and median (Q_Λ) edge sharpness of the porcine models p_1 and p_2 at the heart phase $\phi_3 \approx 30$ % . The best values are marked in bold.

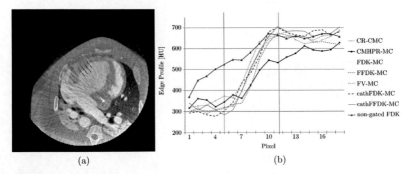

(a)   (b)

Figure 4.22: Measurements of the edge response profile for the porcine model p_1. (a) Visualized lines for edge response function and sharpness for the porcine model p_1. (b) Mean edge response profile for porcine dataset p_1 of the different motion compensation algorithms at 30 % heart phase.

4.7   First Clinical Patient Data

For a first clinical patient dataset, image acquisition was performed using an Artis zeego system (Siemens AG, Healthcare Sector, Forchheim, Germany). The imaging and contrast protocol of the previously presented porcine models [De B 13b, Mlle 13d] needed to be adapted due to the clinical applicability. The acquisition time was 14 s capturing 381 projection images with 26 f/s, and an angular increment of 0.52° during one C-arm rotation. The isotropic pixel resolution was 0.31 mm/pixel (0.19 mm in isocenter) and the detector size was 1240 × 960 pixel. The heart rate was stimulated through external heart pacing to 115 bpm, which is lower as the frequency used for the porcine models (131 bpm). Furthermore, the pacing was performed in the right ventricle instead of the right atrium due to the facilitation of the clinical workflow. Due to the lower pacing frequency, no strict gating was performed, since this would have limited the number of projection images per heart phase to 27. Therefore, the width of the gating window was set to $w = 10$ %, resulting in 34 projections available for reconstruction of each heart phase. For this dataset, a number of $K = 10$ volumes were reconstructed, each at a relative heart phase between 0 % and 100 % with an increment of 10 %. A volume of 91 ml undiluted contrast agent fluid was administered in the pulmonary artery at a speed of 7 ml/s beginning 13 s before the X-ray rotation was started. The X-ray delay was determined by a test bolus injection. Image reconstruction was performed on an image volume of $(25.6 \text{ cm})^3$ distributed on a 256^3 voxel grid. The cathFDK-MC reconstruction results are presented in Figure 4.23 for a systolic and diastolic heart phase. It can be seen that the catheter and pacing electrode still degrade the final image quality, hence, a motion-compensated reconstruction can be performed with the catheter removed projection images, denoted as cathFDK-MC$_{\text{CAR}}$. The initial cathFDK reconstructions and the resulting cathFDK-MC$_{\text{CAR}}$ reconstructions are presented in Figure 4.24 for a systolic and diastolic heart phase, respectively.

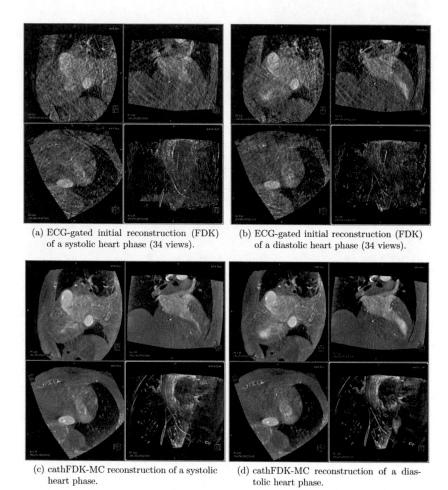

(a) ECG-gated initial reconstruction (FDK)
of a systolic heart phase (34 views).

(b) ECG-gated initial reconstruction (FDK)
of a diastolic heart phase (34 views).

(c) cathFDK-MC reconstruction of a systolic
heart phase.

(d) cathFDK-MC reconstruction of a diastolic heart phase.

Figure 4.23: First results of a clinical patient dataset with the cathFDK-MC reconstruction
of a systolic ($\approx 60\pm3\,\%$) and end-diastolic ($\approx 3\pm1\,\%$) heart phase (W 2080 HU, C 110 HU,
slice thickness 1 mm). The image data was provided by Dr. med. Abt and Dr. med. Köhler
from the Herz- und Kreislaufzentrum Rotenburg a. d. Fulda, Germany.

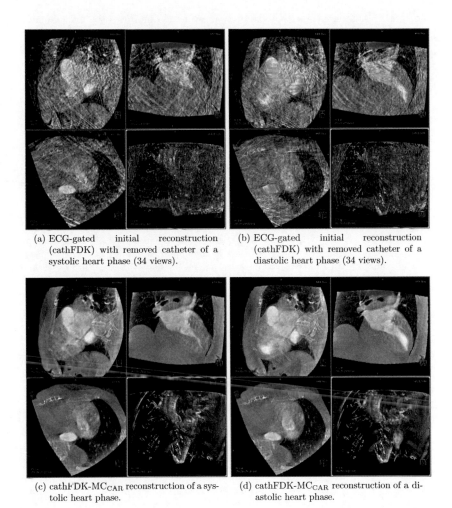

(a) ECG-gated initial reconstruction (cathFDK) with removed catheter of a systolic heart phase (34 views).

(b) ECG-gated initial reconstruction (cathFDK) with removed catheter of a diastolic heart phase (34 views).

(c) cathFDK-MC$_{CAR}$ reconstruction of a systolic heart phase.

(d) cathFDK-MC$_{CAR}$ reconstruction of a diastolic heart phase.

Figure 4.24: First results of a clinical patient dataset with the cathFDK-MC reconstruction and interpolated projection images of a systolic ($\approx$60$\pm$3 %) and end-diastolic ($\approx$3$\pm$1 %) heart phase (W 2080 HU, C 110 HU, slice thickness 1 mm). The image data was provided by Dr. med. Abt and Dr. med. Köhler from the Herz- und Kreislaufzentrum Rotenburg a. d. Fulda, Germany.

4.8   Challenges

The presented results show that the motion estimation improves the image quality compared to the initial images. The extent to which the motion vector fields can represent not only the cardiac wall motion but also the motion of other structures, e.g., like the valves must be evaluated. The motion of the heart valves follows a different motion pattern compared to the endocardial wall motion.

Furthermore, the recently developed acquisition and contrast protocol [De B 13b], which was used in all studies, shows very promising results on the porcine models. In the clinical application, it provides some challenges. If multiple 3-D cardiac images are used for identification and localization of wall motion pathologies, no artificial contraction behavior of the heart is desirable. Hence, the placement of the pacing electrode is critical. Therefore, right atrial pacing would be the place of choice. However, placing the electrode inside the right atrium and getting in contact with the atrial wall is more complicated than placing it inside the right ventricular apex. The influence of the pacing either inside the right atrium or in the right ventricle on the heart physiology needs to be evaluated.

Furthermore, in clinical routine, it is not practical to raise the patient's arms above the head for the whole procedure [Ecto 09]. Consequently, a higher absorption occurs in the lateral projections, caused by the superposition of the arms and the thorax. This leads to a degradation of the image quality in the lateral images and consequently, inconsistent projection data.

The contrast protocol is also challenging, in order to get a sufficient contrast inside the heart chambers and to keep the amount of contrast agent to a minimum. The contrast administration starts before the imaging. Therefore, a test bolus injection is performed before the 3-D image acquisition to determine the X-ray delay required to ensure that the heart chambers are filled with contrast. The timing needs to be identified precisely during the test bolus injection. If the timing is off target, no contrast is present inside the chambers for the first couple of projections. This yields again inconsistent projection data.

4.9   Summary and Conclusions

In this chapter, different volume-based motion estimation algorithms were presented and evaluated for a recently presented one sweep C-arm acquisition protocol. The initial volumes are all based on retrospective ECG-gating to reconstruct multiple heart phases. For this approach, in order to estimate cardiac motion, a longer imaging time is used and, hence, the number of projection images increases compared to the acquisition protocol used in Chapter 3. The ECG-gated reconstructions (FDK) delineate the endocardial boundaries, but the image quality is still degraded by streak artifacts and noise. As an image enhancement step, a bilateral filter was applied to the initial ECG-gated volumes (FFDK) to eliminate noise while preserving the sharp endocardial boundaries. For this application, a pacing electrode and a catheter are always present in the scanning field of view, and cause severe streak artifacts in the ECG-gated reconstructions. Thus, dense objects, i.e. the catheter and the pacing electrode need to be segmented (cathFDK) before the reconstruction step. An additional bilateral filter can be applied on the catheter removed ECG-gated reconstructions (cathFFDK). Initial images were also reconstructed with a few-view iterative reconstruction technique (FV), here the prior image constrained compressed sensing (PICCS) algorithm with the improved total variation (iTV) was used. However, the resulting volumes have a smoother appearance than a standard non-gated FDK reconstruction.

Since the initial image quality is not sufficient, three different motion estimation techniques were compared to each other. The first approach, cardiac registration with cyclic constraints (CR-CMC) represents the cardiac motion by a dense motion vector field and introduces cyclic constraints into the registration framework. The original algorithm was adapted from respiratory motion estimation presented in Brehm et al. [Breh 12]. Here, the CR-CMC was directly applied to the ECG-gated reconstructions. The second algorithm, the 3-D/4-D combined multiple heart phase registration (CMHPR) deforms the sum of the ECG-gated volumes to fit to a reference volume. The reference volume was reconstructed with the prior image constrained compressed sensing (PICCS) algorithm with the improved total variation (iTV). The last motion estimation technique called D-CR performs the motion estimation individually between two heart phases. The 3-D/3-D deformable cardiac registration (D-CR) method uses a deformable B-Spline model to represent the cardiac motion. For this approach, all previously mentioned initial images were evaluated with respect to the final motion-compensated reconstruction quality.

All three motion estimation algorithms were tested on two simulated phantom datasets, with and without a catheter, and two porcine models. For the phantom data the 3-D normalized (nRMSE) and relative root mean square error (rRMSE) and the universal image quality index (UQI) were computed. In addition, for the phantoms, the endocardial sharpness and accuracy of the motion-compensated algorithms were evaluated compared to the gold standard reconstruction without motion. For the two porcine models, the sharpness of the endocardium was measured in a systolic heart phase. In general, all motion-compensated reconstructions improved the image quality compared to the initial volume data. The overall quantitative results show that if no dense object is present in the field of view, the D-CR algorithm independent of the initial images and the CR-CMC outperform the CMHPR approach. The CMHPR motion-compensated reconstruction improves the image quality compared to the ECG-gated reconstructions. However, if the endocardial borders of the reference reconstruction are already blurred during the iterative reconstruction, the CMHPR cannot recover the sharp edges. For the phantom data with a catheter and the two porcine models, the D-CR approach on initial images where the catheter and pacing electrode were removed before the motion estimation step and and the CR-CMC achieve the best results. For future investigations, different initial images for the CR-CMC and CMHPR registrations should be considered.

The first patient dataset results are quite promising and indicate that the motion estimation and compensation approaches can be applied to a broader database in clinical practice.

CHAPTER 5

Summary and Outlook

5.1 Summary. 125

5.2 Outlook 128

5.1 Summary

In this thesis, algorithmic concepts for dynamic three-dimensional tomographic imaging of the heart chambers using an interventional C-arm CT system have been presented. C-arm systems are the main imaging modality in interventional cardiac imaging. In general, 2-D fluoroscopic images are acquired during the procedure for analysis, diagnosis and guidance. Additionally, these systems provide the possibility to acquire 2-D X-ray images while rotating around the patient. These images can be used for a 3-D tomographic reconstruction. For 3-D cardiac imaging with an angiographic C-arm system, the acquisition time of a rotational scan lasts several seconds and thus, covers several heart cycles. The acquired data contains the complete dynamic of the heart and thus, requires new reconstruction techniques that consider these dynamics. The cardiac motion has to be estimated and compensated. Therefore, the main focus of this thesis lies in the development of new advanced motion estimation and compensation techniques for 3-D cardiac imaging using interventional C-arm systems. Two approaches have been investigated in this thesis. They are based on the surface or on the volume of the heart chambers. The approaches require different image acquisition protocols which must be included in the assessment.

A short introduction into the cardiac anatomy and the cardiac cycle has been given in Chapter 1. Furthermore, the clinical relevance of interventional three-dimensional cardiac imaging has been explained in comparison to other modalities used for cardiac imaging. In particular, the differences between C-arm CT and conventional CT have been highlighted. The chapter concludes with the summary of the scientific contribution of the presented work to the progress of research.

Chapter 2 comprises state-of-the-art techniques focusing on the cardiac chamber and cardiovascular image reconstruction techniques. Most techniques map the reconstruction problem of dynamic objects to the reconstruction formulation of static objects. The most popular approach utilizes an electrocardiogram (ECG) signal acquired synchronously with the acquisition in order to use only the projection data belonging to a certain motion state. This results in a sparse angular sampling of the available projection data, which then leads to a low signal to noise ratio, severe streak artifacts and low-contrast structures that cannot be reliably resolved. The amount of undersampling is dependent on the specific acquisition protocol, the heart rate of the patient and the imaging framerate. In recent years, many constrained iterative image reconstruction approaches (often denoted as compressed sensing) using different imaging cost functions in order to increase image quality have been proposed. However, the image quality and visual impression varies tremendously with the parameter selection and regularization weighting and often results in an over-smoothed and piecewise constant image impression. Another technique is the estimation of the motion and the utilization of all the acquired projection data in terms of a motion compensated reconstruction algorithm. The use of all projection images significantly increases the signal-to-noise ratio compared to the retrospective ECG-gated images. However, the motion estimation step is the crucial and challenging part. Volume-based approaches require a reference image and initial images of sufficiently good image quality. The generation of initial 3-D images from one rotation of a C-arm that are useful for motion estimation by deformable registration is quite challenging. Consequently, motion estimation techniques from other modalities, e.g., CT cannot be directly applied to the C-arm CT data.

Algorithms specifically developed for cardiac vasculature reconstruction deploy different assumptions which do not hold for cardiac chambers. The chambers differ from the sparse and high contrast structure of the coronary arteries, hence, some pre-processing steps assuming sparse and high contrast objects are not feasible. Furthermore, a larger number of projection images are required for a retrospective ECG-gated reconstruction of a non-sparse object, like the cardiac chambers.

Two individual approaches have been developed with respect to the respective clinical application and available image data. The first approach utilizes extracted surface models and can be used for a one chamber visualization and reconstruction, e.g., of the left ventricle. The second approach works on initially reconstructed volumes and provides the possibility to reconstruct two or four cardiac chambers. However, the volume-based approach requires a longer scan time, more contrast agent and a higher dose.

In Chapter 3, a complete framework for left ventricular tomographic reconstruction and wall motion analysis has been presented. Dynamic surface models were generated from the 2-D X-ray images acquired during a short scan of a C-arm scanner using the 2-D bloodpool information. The acquisition time was 5 s and the patient showed a normal sinus rhythm. Due to the slow rotation speed of the C-arm, no valuable retrospective ECG-gated reconstructions were possible. The dynamic surface LV model comprises a sparse motion vector field on the surface, but in order to perform a tomographic motion-compensated reconstruction, a dense motion vector field is required. Therefore, the influence of different motion interpolation methods was investigated. A thin-plate spline, Shepard's method, a smoothed weighting based approach and simple averaging were used. The best quantitative results, based on the Dice coefficient and the mean contour deviation, for a phantom, a porcine, and three human datasets were achieved using the TPS interpolation approach. Shepard's method and the smoothed weighting function might be a good compromise between computational efficiency and accuracy. The framework also enables the analysis of the contraction behavior of the LV via the surface model. Functional parameters, e.g., ejection fraction and systolic dyssynchrony index known from other modalities were transferred to C-arm CT data. A feasibility study on simulated phantom LVs with pathological defects as well as on eight clinical datasets indicate the capability of the presented framework. The dynamic surface model together with a colored overlay of the contraction activity in 3-D might provide additional clinically useful information. The combination of the wall motion analysis with the motion-compensated reconstruction is of great value to the diagnosis of pathological regions in cardiac interventions. In conclusion, the first framework which enables LV wall motion analysis directly in the catheter lab during a cardiac intervention using intra-procedural C-arm CT data was presented.

In Chapter 4, a different problem has been addressed, where two or four chambers shall be reconstructed. Due to the overlap of the chambers, surface-based methods fail in the 2D segmentation step of the projection images. Therefore, different volume-based motion estimation algorithms have been presented and evaluated for a recently presented one sweep C-arm acquisition protocol. A longer acquisition time is required to allow for retrospective ECG-gating of non-sparse objects to reconstruct multiple heart phases. The ECG-gated reconstructions delineate the endocardial boundaries, but the image quality is degraded by streak artifacts and noise. Since the initial image quality achieved with the previously mentioned techniques is not sufficient, motion estimation and compensation methods are required. Additionally, the image quality of the initial images needs to be improved in order to estimate the cardiac motion reliably. As an image enhancement step, a bilateral filter has been applied to the initial ECG-gated volumes to eliminate noise while preserving the sharp endocardial boundaries. Due to the clinical acquisition protocol, a pacing electrode and a catheter filled with contrast agent are always present in the scanning field of view. Hence, they cause severe streak artifacts in the ECG-gated reconstructions. Thus, those dense objects need to be segmented and removed before the reconstruction. An additional bilateral filter has been applied on the catheter removed ECG-gated reconstructions. Furthermore, initial images have been reconstructed with a few-view iterative reconstruction technique, here the prior image constrained compressed sensing (PICCS) algorithm with the improved total variation (iTV) has been used. However, the resulting volumes have a smoother appearance than a standard non-gated FDK reconstruction. Three different motion estimation techniques have been compared to each other. The first approach, the cardiac registration with cyclic motion constraints (CR-CMC) represents the cardiac motion by a dense motion vector field and introduces cyclic constraints into the registration framework. The original algorithm has been adapted from respiratory motion estimation presented in Brehm et al. [Breh 12]. Here, the CR-CMC was directly applied to the ECG-gated reconstructions. The second algorithm, the 3-D/4-D combined multiple heart phase registration (CMHPR) approach deforms the sum of the ECG-gated volumes to fit to a reference volume. The reference volume was reconstructed with the prior image constrained compressed sensing (PICCS) algorithm with the improved total variation (iTV). The last motion estimation technique called 3-D/3-D deformable cardiac registration (D-CR) performs the motion estimation individually between two heart phases. The D-CR method uses a deformable B-Spline model to represent the cardiac motion.

All three volume-based motion estimation algorithms were tested on two simulated phantom datasets, with and without a catheter, and two porcine models. The overall quantitative results show that if no dense object is present in the field of view, the D-CR algorithm and the CR-CMC outperform the CMHPR approach. The CMHPR motion-compensated reconstruction improves the image quality compared to the ECG-gated reconstructions. However, if the endocardial borders of the reference reconstruction are already blurred during the iterative reconstruction, the CMHPR cannot recover sharp edges. For the phantom data with a catheter and the two porcine models, the D-CR approach on initial images where the catheter and pacing electrode have been removed before the motion estimation step achieves the best results. For future investigations, different initial images for the CR-CMC and CMHPR registrations should also be considered.

The first patient dataset results are quite promising and indicate that the motion estimation and compensation approaches can be applied to a broader database in clinical practice.

5.2 Outlook

This thesis provides approaches and solutions for interventional cardiac chamber reconstructions using C-arm CT data. The results bring interventional cardiac chamber imaging closer to the daily clinical routine to support complex cardiac procedures and interventional diagnosis. For the left ventricular surface-based motion estimation and compensation method, not only can the motion, extracted from the generated surface models, be used for analysis of ventricular wall motion, but also the computed dense motion vector fields can be used to physiologically analyze the cardiac motion. Additionally, wall motion analysis can also be performed with the motion vector fields, estimated from the volume-based approach. Up to now, cardiac functional analysis in the catheterization lab is not well developed. During the intervention, quantitative measurements are limited to 2-D fluoroscopic images. The results of this thesis created a basis to provide additional functional parameters — such as wall thickening, fractional shortening, phase of contraction or dyssynchrony index — directly to an interventional setting.

As discussed before, the volume-based 3-D reconstructions are challenging due to the heart motion which necessitates high temporal resolution. Multi-segment retrospective ECG-gating can be applied to reconstruct 3-D images of different cardiac phases and different image enhancement techniques can be applied to improve the initial image quality. In a second step, the motion between these phases can be estimated using deformable image registration. The deformation fields found in this manner are a crucial step for an accurate and precise motion-compensated reconstruction. Various representations of motion, e.g., B-splines, thin-plate splines or dense motion vector fields can be used. Therefore, the influence of the different models can be studied in more detail with respect to the resulting motion vector fields. Additionally, there exist many different objective functions and regularization techniques in the field of deformable medical image registration. These can be exploited with respect to cardiac motion, since the results of this thesis show that it is possible to estimate cardiac motion from preprocessed images.

List of Abbreviations and Symbols

Abbreviations

3DE   Three-dimensional Echocardiography 5

3DFS   Three-dimensional Fractional Shortening 45

cathFDK   Catheter-removed ECG-gated FDK Reconstruction 80

cathFDK-MC   Motion compensation using D-CR with cathFDK 92

cathFFDK   Bilateral-filtered and Catheter-removed ECG-gated FDK Recon. 82

cathFFDK-MC Motion compensation using D-CR and cathFFDK 92

CCTA   Cardiac Computed Tomography Angiography 35

CMHPR   Combined Multiple Heart Phase Registration 88

CMHPR-MC   Motion-compensated Reconstruction using CMHPR 92

CR-CMC   Cardiac Registration with Cyclic Motion Constraints 85

CRT   Cardiac Resynchronization Therapy 35

CS   Compressed Sensing 20

CT   Computed Tomography 6

D-CR   Deformable Cardiac Registration 90

DRR   Digitally Reconstructed Radiograph 18

DSC   Dice Similarity Coefficient 50

ECG   Electrocardiogram 12

ED   End-diastolic 36

EDV   End-diastolic Volume 44

EF   Ejection Fraction 44

ES   End-systolic 36

ESV   End-systolic Volume 44

FBP   Filtered-backprojection 17

FDK   ECG-gated FDK Reconstruction 79

FDK   Feldkamp, Davis and Kress Algorithm 11

FDK-MC   Motion compensation using D-CR with FDK 92

FDK-MC   Motion compensation using D-CR with FFDK 92

FFDK   Bilateral-filtered ECG-gated FDK Reconstruction 80

FV   Iterative Few-view Reconstruction 84

FV-MC   Motion compensation using D-CR with FV 92

ICE   Intracardiac Echocardiography 5

iTV   Improved Total Variation 21

LV   Left Ventricle 23

MIP   Maximum Intensity Projection 50

MRI   Magnetic Resonance Imaging 6

MVF   Motion Vector Field 34

NCC   Normalized Cross Correlation 88

nRMSE   Normalized Root Mean Square Error 48

PBT   Probabilistic Boosting Tree 36

PCA   Principal Component Analysis 43

PET   Positron Emission Tomography 7

PICCS   Prior Image Constrained Compressed Sensing 20

ROI   Region of Interest 49

rRMSE   relative Root Mean Square Error 103

SDI   Systolic Dyssynchrony Index 45

SNR   Signal-to-Noise-Ratio 20

SPECT   Single Positron Emission Tomography 7

SSD   Sum of Squared Differences 26

SVD   Singular Value Decomposition 42

TAVI   Transcatheter Aortic Valve Implantation 76

TEE	Transesophageal Echocardiography	5
TPS	Thin-plate Spline	39
TTE	Transthoracic Echocardiography	5
TV	Total Variation	21
UQI	Universal Image Quality Index	48
US	Ultrasound	26

Symbols

α PICCS weighting parameter 21

$\boldsymbol{A} \in \mathbb{R}^{3\times3}$ affine transformation matrix (rotation, shearing and scaling) . . 39

$\boldsymbol{b} \in \mathbb{R}^3$ translation vector 39

$\boldsymbol{c}$ thin-plate spline coefficients $\in \mathbb{R}^{3P_c}$ 39

$\boldsymbol{d}$ motion vector at $\boldsymbol{x} \in \mathbb{R}^3$ 38

$\boldsymbol{d}_c$ motion vector defined at surface control point $\boldsymbol{p}_c \in \mathbb{R}^3$ 38

$\boldsymbol{n}_1, \boldsymbol{n}_2, \boldsymbol{n}_3$ local LV coordinate system 43

$\boldsymbol{p}_c$ surface control point $\in \mathbb{R}^3$ 38

$\boldsymbol{s}$ vector of real valued parameters $\in \mathbb{R}^{K_S}$ 16

$\boldsymbol{s}_{\text{Data}}$ function parameters of the data consistency optimized object . . 21

$\boldsymbol{s}_{\text{im}}$ image basis function parameters 18

$\boldsymbol{s}_{\text{Sparse}}$ function parameters of the TV optimized object 22

$\boldsymbol{s}_{\text{ga}}$ gating parameter vector, $\boldsymbol{s}_{\text{ga}} = (\phi_r, w, \vartheta)^T$ 24

$\boldsymbol{s}_{\text{mm}}$ motion vector parameter $\in \mathbb{R}^{K_{\text{mm}}}$ 29

$\boldsymbol{u}$ pixel coordinate $\in \mathbb{R}^2$ 16

$\boldsymbol{x}$ voxel coordinate $\in \mathbb{R}^3$ 16

Δ mean edge sharpness measure for phantom data 103

ϵ data consistency error 21

ϵ_p average point-to-mesh error 65

$\epsilon_{\mathcal{C}}$ mean contour deviation 52

η iTV step width in 3-D 22

Λ mean edge sharpness measure for porcine data 104

λ gating function returning the weight of the i-th image 24

λ_c euclidean distance from every surface point to long axis 45

$\overline{\pi}$ reference time-size 2-D bloodpool function 36

ϕ function returning the relative heart phase $\in [0,1]$ 23

ϕ_k discrete heart phase number, with $k = 1, \ldots, K$ 24

ϕ_r	reference heart phase	24
$\phi_{c,\max}$	heart phase to maximal contraction for surface point $\boldsymbol{p}_c$	45
$\phi_{s,\max}$	heart phase to maximal contraction for segment s	45
Π	3-D LV volume function	44
π	2-D bloodpool function	36
π_f	smoothed 2-D bloodpool function	36
π_n	normalized 2-D bloodpool function	37
Ψ	sparsity transform	20
ψ	intermediate heart phase $\psi \in [0,1]$	36
τ	mean edge error measure for phantom data	104
ε	singularity avoidance parameter	21
ϑ	gating window form	24
$\tilde{\boldsymbol{s}}_{\mathrm{mm}}$	motion parameters between reference and current phase, $\in \mathbb{R}^{\widetilde{K}_{\mathrm{mm}}}$	38
$\widetilde{K}_{\mathrm{mm}}$	number of motion parameters between ref. and current phase	38
A	system matrix function	19
B	perspective projection operator from 3-D to 2-D	17
C	geometrical scaling constant	18
c	function for cosine and redundancy weighting	17
D	number of data consistency iterations	22
d	dissimilarity (distance) measure	20
d_ϕ	closeness function between two heart phases	23
F	number of TV optimization iterations	22
f	function that provides access to the reconstructed values in 3-D	16
f_{Data}	function provides access to the data consistency object in 3-D	21
f_{Sparse}	function provides access to the TV optimized object in 3-D	22
f_P	function that provides access to values of the prior image in 3-D	21
$f_{\phi_k,f}$	bilateral filtered reconstruction function	80
f_{ϕ_k}	function that provides access to values of ECG-gated volume	26

g row-wise filtering kernel 18

h_{FDK} i-th distance-weighted and pre-processed projection value 17

I center of rotation 16

i projection image number $i = 1, \dots, N$ 17

K number of heart phases 24

K_s number of elements of $\boldsymbol{s}$ 16

K_{mm} number of motion vector parameters 29

l linear interpolation parameter 40

$L_{i,\boldsymbol{u}}$ measurement ray for projection i and pixel $\boldsymbol{u}$ 19

M motion model function 29

m side length of 2-D projection image 93

N number of projection images 17

n side length of 3-D volume 42

n_c linear interpolation parameter: number of points 40

O outer iterations for constrained iterative reconstruction 22

p pre-processed projection data function (line integrals) 18

P_c number of surface control points 38

p_F pre-processed, filtered and redundancy weighted projection fct. . 17

R linear interpolation parameter: radius 40

r function which provides access to the DRR value in 2-D 19

r_c region of interest for motion estimation 41

r_f filter size 93

S X-ray source 16

S_L number of multi-resolution scales 94

S_w number of forward and backward runs 25

s_w current C-arm sweep $s_w \in 1, \dots, S_w$ 25

T number of iterative MVF corrections 94

u linear weighting function 40

W number of registration iterations 94

w gating window width 24

w_{iTV} iTV step width in 2-D 22

w_D distance weight function of FDK formula 17

$\mathcal{B}_{\mathrm{FW}}, \mathcal{B}_{\mathrm{GS}}$ binary mask 2-D images 50

$\mathcal{C}_{\mathrm{FW}}, \mathcal{C}_{\mathrm{GS}}$ contour binary 2-D images 50

$\mathcal{N}$ subset of projection images 20

$3\mathrm{DFS}_c$ three-dimensional fractional shortening for point c 45

List of Figures

1.1 Heart anatomy 2
1.2 Heart anatomy in MRI image 3
1.3 Temporal correlation of left ventricular pressure, volume and ECG-signal 4
1.4 Heart anatomy in CT image 5
1.5 Example of C-arm CT systems 9

2.1 C-arm CT geometry 17
2.2 Perspective projection mappings 19
2.3 Schematic overview of the improved total variation (iTV) algorithm . 22
2.4 Example of ECG-gated reconstruction of a left ventricle from a 5 s scan. 24
2.5 Scheme of motion compensation 30
2.6 ECG-gated reconstruction of a left ventricle and a left coronary artery 31

3.1 Schematic overview of Chapter 3 34
3.2 Cardiac phase identification 37
3.3 Example of an extracted surface model & sparse Motion vector field . 39
3.4 Thin-plate spline motion vector fields based on surface models 42
3.5 Representation of left ventricle for motion analysis 44
3.6 Dynamic FDK and static reconstruction of the ventricle phantom dataset 49
3.7 Contour projections for motion-compensated reconstruction quality . 51
3.8 Surface-based motion-compensated reconstructions of the phantom . 55
3.9 Surface-based motion-compensated reconstruction results of porcine . 56
3.10 Surface-based motion-compensated reconstruction of dataset h_1 . . . 57
3.11 Reconstructions of dataset h_1 with different interpolation schemes . . 58
3.12 Examples of the GT phantom models and surface models 61
3.13 3-D LV volume curves of the different phantoms ($p_{1,\mathrm{GT}}$–$p_{5,\mathrm{GT}}$). 61
3.14 GT Hammer maps of $\phi_{c,\mathrm{max}}$ of the phantom datasets. 63
3.15 GT Hammer maps of 3DFS$_c$ of the phantom datasets. 64
3.16 Correlation of heart phase identification 66
3.17 Estimated Hammer maps of $\phi_{c,\mathrm{max}}$ of the phantom datasets 68
3.18 Difference Hammer maps of $\phi_{c,\mathrm{max}}$ of the phantom datasets 69
3.19 Estimated Hammer maps of 3DFS$_c$ of the phantom datasets 69
3.20 Difference Hammer maps of 3DFS$_c$ of the phantom datasets 70
3.21 Example of surface meshes from clinical data and volume curves . . . 71
3.22 Hammer map $\phi_{c,\mathrm{max}}$ and 3DFS$_c$ for the clinical dataset h_8. 72

4.1 Schematic overview of Chapter 4 78
4.2 Example images of initial ECG-gated reconstructions 79
4.3 Example images of initial bilateral filtered ECG-gated reconstructions 81
4.4 Schematic overview of the catheter removal procedure. 81
4.5 Example images of initial catheter removed ECG-gated reconstructions 83

4.6   Example images of cath. removed & filtered ECG-gated reconstructions 84
4.7   Example images of initial few-view reconstructions 84
4.8   Example images of initial ECG and few-view reconstruction 85
4.9   Overview of the cardiac registration with cyclic motion constraints . . 86
4.10 Overview of the 3-D/4-D combined multiple heart phase registration . 88
4.11 Registration pyramid for B-spline registration. 99
4.12 Example images of the simulated phantom datasets 101
4.13 Central slice of the static phantom and the dynamic phantom 105
4.14 Central slice reconstructions of dynamic phantom without catheter . 107
4.15 Central slice of reconstructions of the phantom with catheter 111
4.16 Edge response profile for the catheter phantom 113
4.17 Axial central slice of reconstructions of p_1 at a heart phase of 30 % . . 114
4.18 Axial central slice of reconstructions of p_1 at a heart phase of 80 % . . 115
4.19 Axial central slice of reconstructions of p_2 at a heart phase of 20 % . . 116
4.20 Axial central slice of reconstructions of p_2 at a heart phase of 80 % . . 117
4.21 Illustration of different heart phases of porcine model p_1 118
4.22 Mean edge profile for porcine model p_1 119
4.23 Results of the first clinical patient dataset 120
4.24 First clinical patient reconstructions with interpolated projections . . 121

List of Tables

1.1   Difference between conventional CT and C-arm CT   9

3.1   Physiological parameters for motion estimation and compensation . .   48
3.2   The nRMSE and UQI of phantom p_0   53
3.3   Dice coefficient and mean contour deviation of phantom p_0   53
3.4   Dice coefficient and mean contour deviation of porcine p_{por}   54
3.5   Dice coefficient and mean contour deviation of patient h_1–h_3   54
3.6   Contraction times of affected GT phantom segments   62
3.7   Parameters of the GT phantom datasets   62
3.8   Point-to-mesh error for phantom surface meshes   65
3.9   Accuracy and Correlation of heart phase identification   66
3.10 Contraction times of affected segments between estimated and GT . .   67
3.11 Results for estimated surface meshes and deviation to GT   68
3.12 Estimated physiological data parameters for clinical datasets   71
3.13 Rotation angle variation of the clinical datasets.   71

4.1   Complexity analysis of the initial image reconstructions   94
4.2   Complexity analysis of the different motion estimation algorithms. . .   94
4.3   Overview of the different generated phantoms   100
4.4   Quantitative results of dynamic phantom model without catheter . .   106
4.5   Mean edge sharpness deviation Δ of the phantom model without catheter   108
4.6   Mean error τ of the edge profile of the phantom without catheter . .   108
4.7   Quantitative results of the phantom model with the catheter   110
4.8   Mean edge sharpness deviation Δ of the phantom model with catheter   112
4.9   Mean error τ of the edge profile of the phantom with catheter   112
4.10 Mean edge sharpness Λ of the porcine models   118

List of Algorithms

4.1   Combined Multiple Heart Phase Registration (CMHPR).   97
4.2   Objective function and derivative computation.   98

Bibliography

[Abba 13]   S. Abbas, T. Lee, S. Shin, R. Lee, and S. Cho. "Effects of sparse sampling schemes on image quality in low-dose CT". *Medical Physics*, Vol. 40, No. 11, pp. 111915-1–12, November 2013.

[Ache 06]   S. Achenbach, D. Ropers, A. Kuettner, T. Flohr, B. Ohnesorge, H. Bruder, H. Theessen, M. Karakaya, W. G. Daniel, W. Bautz, W. A. Kalender, and K. Anders. "Contrast-enhanced coronary artery visualization by dual-source computed tomography - Initial experience". *European Journal of Radiology*, Vol. 57, No. 3, pp. 331–335, March 2006.

[Ache 09]   S. Achenbach, M. Marwan, T. Schepis, T. Pflederer, H. Bruder, T. Allmendinger, M. Petersilka, K. Anders, M. Lell, A. Kuettner, D. Ropers, W. G. Daniel, and T. Flohr. "High-pitch spiral acquisition: a new scan mode for coronary CT angiography". *Journal of Cardiovascular Computed Tomography*, Vol. 3, No. 2, pp. 117–121, March 2009.

[Al A 08]   A. Al-Ahmad, L. Wigström, D. Sandner-Porkristl, P. J. Wang, P. C. Zei, J. Boese, G. Lauritsch, T. Moore, F. Chan, and R. Fahrig. "Time-resolved three-dimensional imaging of the left atrium and pulmonary veins in the interventional suite–a comparison between multisweep gated rotational three-dimensional reconstructed fluoroscopy and multislice computed tomography". *Heart Rhythm*, Vol. 5, No. 4, pp. 513–519, April 2008.

[Back 05]   W. Backfrieder, M. Carpella, R. Swoboda, C. Steinwender, C. Gabriel, and F. Leisch. "Model Based LV-Reconstruction in Bi-Plane X-ray Angiography". In: J. Fitzpatrick and J. Reinhardt, Eds., *Proceedings of SPIE Medical Imaging 2005: Image Processing. February 12-18, 2005, San Diego, CA, USA*. pp. 1475–1483.

[Bart 13]   T. Bartel, S. Müller, A. Biviano, and R. T. Hahn. "Why is intracardiac echocardiography helpful? Benefits, costs, and how to learn". *European Heart Journal*, Vol. 35, No. 2, pp. 69–76, October 2013.

[Beck 09]   C. Becker, R. Loose, O. Meißner, and M. Reiser. "C-Bogen-CT - ein Meilenstein der interventionellen Bildgebung". *Der Radiologe*, Vol. 49, No. 9, p. 810, September 2009.

[Bian 10]   J. Bian, J. Siewerdsen, X. Han, E. Y. Sidky, J. L. Prince, C. A. Pelizzari, and X. Pan. "Evaluation of sparse-view reconstruction from flat-panel-detector cone-beam CT". *Physics in Medicine and Biology*, Vol. 55, No. 22, pp. 6575–6599, October 2010.

[Blon 04]   C. Blondel, R. Vaillant, G. Malandain, and N. Ayache. "3D tomographic reconstruction of coronary arteries using a precomputed 4D motion field". *Physics in Medicine and Biology*, Vol. 49, No. 11, pp. 2197–2208, June 2004.

[Blon 06]   C. Blondel, G. Malandain, R. Vaillant, and N. Ayache. "Reconstruction of Coronary Arteries from a Single Rotational X-Ray Projection

Sequence". *IEEE Transactions on Medical Imaging*, Vol. 25, No. 5, pp. 653–663, May 2006.

[Blum 10] M. Blume, A. Martinez-Möller, A. Keil, N. Navab, and M. Rafecas. "Joint Reconstruction of Image and Motion in Gated Positron-Emission-Tomography". *IEEE Transactions on Medical Imaging*, Vol. 29, No. 11, pp. 1892–1906, November 2010.

[Boyd 04] S. Boyd and L. Vandenberghe. *Convex Optimization*. Cambridge University Press, 7 Ed., 2004.

[Breh 12] M. Brehm, P. Paysan, M. Oelhafen, P. Kunz, and M. Kachelrieß. "Self-adapting cyclic registration for motion-compensated cone-beam CT in image-guided radiation therapy". *Medical Physics*, Vol. 39, No. 12, pp. 7603–7618, December 2012.

[Breh 13] M. Brehm, P. Paysan, M. Oelhafen, and M. Kachelrieß. "Artifact-resistant motion estimation with a patient-specific artifact model for motion-compensated cone-beam CT". *Medical Physics*, Vol. 40, No. 10, pp. 101913-1–13, October 2013.

[Bros 12] A. Brost, A. Wimmer, R. Liao, F. Bourier, M. Koch, N. Strobel, K. Kurzidim, and J. Hornegger. "Constrained Registration for Motion Compensation in Atrial Fibrillation Ablation Procedures". *IEEE Transactions on Medical Imaging*, Vol. 31, No. 4, pp. 870–881, April 2012.

[Budo 01] M. J. Budoff and P. Raggi. "Coronary artery disease progression assessed by electron-beam computed tomography". *The American Journal of Cardiology*, Vol. 88, No. 2, pp. 46–50, July 2001.

[Budo 06] M. J. Budoff, S. Achenbach, R. Blumenthal, J. J. Carr, J. G. Goldin, P. Greenland, A. D. Guerci, J. A. C. Lima, D. J. Rader, G. D. Rubin, L. J. Shaw, and S. E. Wiegers. "Assessment of Coronary Artery Disease by Cardiac Computed Tomography". *Circulation*, Vol. 114, No. 16, pp. 1761–1791, October 2006.

[Buzu 08] T. Buzug. *Computed Tomography From Photon Statistics to Modern Cone-Beam CT*. Springer Verlag Berlin Heidelberg, 2008 Ed., 2008.

[Cach 99] P. Cachier, X. Pennec, and N. Ayache. "Fast Non Rigid Matching by Gradient Descent: Study and Improvements of the 'Demons' Algorithm". Tech. Rep. 3706, Institut National de Recherche en Informatique et en Automatique (INRIA), June 1999.

[Camm 11] J. Cammin, P. Khurd, A. Kamen, Q. Tang, K. J. Kirchberg, C. Chefd' Hotel, H. Bruder, and K. Taguchi. "Combined Motion Estimation and Motion compensated FBP for Cardiac CT". In: M. Kachelriess and M. Rafecas, Eds., *Proceedings of the 11th International Meeting on Fully Three-Dimensional Image Reconstruction in Radiology and Nuclear Medicine (Fully3D)*. July 11-15, 2011, Potsdam, Germany. pp. 136–139.

[Cand 06a] E. J. Candès. "Compressive Sampling". In: M. Sanz-Solè, J. Varona, J. Soria, and J. Verdera, Eds., *Proceedings of the International Congress of Mathematicians (ICM) 2006*. EMS Publishing House Zürich, *August 22-30, 2006, Madrid, Spain*. pp. 1433–1452.

[Cand 06b]   E. J. Candès, J. Romberg, and T. Tao. "Robust uncertainty principles: exact signal reconstruction from highly incomplete frequency information". *IEEE Transactions on Information Theory*, Vol. 52, No. 2, pp. 489–509, February 2006.

[Cand 07]   E. J. Candès and J. Romberg. "Sparsity and incoherence in compressive sampling". *Inverse Problems*, Vol. 23, No. 3, pp. 969–985, June 2007.

[Cand 08]   E. J. Candès and M. B. Wakin. "An Introduction to Compressive Sampling". *IEEE Signal Processing Magazine*, Vol. 25, No. 2, pp. 21–30, March 2008.

[Cerq 02]   M. D. Cerqueira, N. J. Weissman, V. Dilsizian, A. K. Jacobs, S. Kaul, W. K. Laskey, D. Pennell, J. A. Rumberger, T. Ryan, and A. Verani, M. S. "Standardized myocardial segmentation and nomenclature for tomographic imaging of the heart: a statement for healthcare professionals from the Cardiac Imaging Committee of the Council on Clinical Cardiology of the American Heart Association". *Circulation*, Vol. 105, No. 4, pp. 539–542, January 2002.

[Chen 08]   G.-H. Chen, J. Tang, and S. Leng. "Prior image constrained compressed sensing (PICCS): A method to accurately reconstruct dynamic CT images from highly undersampled projection data sets". *Medical Physics*, Vol. 35, No. 2, pp. 660–663, February 2008.

[Chen 11]   M. Chen, Y. Zheng, K. Müller, C. Rohkohl, G. Lauritsch, J. Boese, G. Funka-Lea, J. Hornegger, and D. Comaniciu. "Automatic Extraction of 3D Dynamic Left Ventricle Model from 2D Rotational Angiocardiogram". In: G. Fichtinger, A. Martel, and T. Peters, Eds., *Proceedings of the Medical Imaging and Computer Assisted Interventions (MICCAI) 2011.* Springer Verlag Berlin Heidelberg, *September 18-22, 2011, Toronto, Canada.* pp. 471–478.

[Chen 12]   G.-H. Chen, P. Thèriault-Lauzier, J. Tang, B. Nett, S. Leng, J. Zambelli, Q. Zhihua, N. Bevins, A. Raval, and S. Reeder. "Time-Resolved Interventional Cardiac C-arm Cone-Beam CT: An Application of the PICCS Algorithm". *IEEE Transactions on Medical Imaging*, Vol. 31, No. 4, pp. 907–923, April 2012.

[Chen 13a]   M. Chen, Y. Zheng, K. Müller, C. Rohkohl, G. Lauritsch, J. Boese, G. Funka-Lea, and D. Comaniciu. "Left Ventricle Epicardium Estimation in Medical Diagnostic Imaging". January 2013. Patent No. US 2013/0004040 A1.

[Chen 13b]   M. Chen, Y. Zheng, K. Müller, C. Rohkohl, G. Lauritsch, J. Boese, G. Funka-Lea, and D. Comaniciu. "Subtraction of Projection Data in Medical Diagnostic Imaging". January 2013. Patent No. 2013/0004052 A1.

[Chen 13c]   M. Chen, Y. Zheng, Y. Wang, K. Müller, and G. Lauritsch. "Automatic 3D Motion Estimation of Left Ventricle from C-arm Rotational Angiocardiography Using a Prior Motion Model and Learning Based Boundary Detector". In: K. Mori, I. Sakuma, Y. Sato, C. Barillot, and N. Navab, Eds., *Proceedings of the Medical Imaging and Computer Assisted Interventions (MICCAI) 2013.* Springer Verlag Berlin Heidelberg, *September 22-26, 2013, Nagoya, Japan.* pp. 90–97.

[Chri 13]   C. P. Christoffersen, D. Hansen, P. Poulsen, and T. S. Sorensen. "Registration-Based Reconstruction of Four-Dimensional Cone Beam Computed Tomography". *IEEE Transactions on Medical Imaging*, Vol. 32, No. 11, pp. 2064–2076, November 2013.

[Chun 09]   S. Y. Chun and J. A. Fessler. "Joint image reconstruction and nonrigid motion estimation with a simple penalty that encourages local invertibility". In: E. Samei and J. Hsieh, Eds., *Proceedings of SPIE Medical Imaging 2009: Physics of Medical Imaging*. February 7-12, 2009, Lake Buena Vista, FL, USA. p. 72580U.

[Daeh 04]   I. Daehnert, C. Rotzsch, M. Wiener, and P. Schneider. "Rapid right ventricular pacing is an alternative to adenosine in catheter interventional procedures for congenital heart disease". *Heart*, Vol. 90, No. 9, pp. 1047–1050, September 2004.

[Davi 13]   B. Davis, K. Royalty, M. Kowarschik, C. Rohkohl, E. Oberstar, B. Aagaard-Kienitz, D. Niemann, O. Ozkan, C. Strother, and C. Mistretta. "4D digital subtraction angiography: implementation and demonstration of feasibility". *American Journal of Neuroradiology*, Vol. 34, No. 10, pp. 1914–1921, April 2013.

[Davi 97]   M. H. Davis, A. Khotanzad, D. P. Flamig, and S. E. Harms. "A Physics-Based Coordinate Transformation for 3-D Image Matching". *IEEE Transactions on Medical Imaging*, Vol. 16, No. 3, pp. 317–328, June 1997.

[De B 13a]   S. De Buck, B. S. Alzand, J.-Y. Wielandts, C. Garweg, T. Phlips, J. Ector, D. Nuyens, and H. Heidbuchel. "Cardiac three-dimensional rotational angiography can be performed with low radiation dose while preserving image quality". *EP Europace*, pp. 1–7, May 2013.

[De B 13b]   S. De Buck, D. Dauwe, J.-Y. Wielandts, P. Claus, C. Koehler, Y. Kyriakou, S. Janssens, H. Heidbuchel, and D. Nuyens. "A new approach for prospectively gated cardiac rotational angiography". In: R. Nishikawa and B. Whiting, Eds., *Proceedings of SPIE Medical Imaging 2013: Physics of Medical Imaging*. February 9-14, 2013, Lake Buena Vista, FL, USA. p. 86682W.

[Deri 87]   R. Deriche. "Using Canny's Criteria to Derive a Recursively Implemented Optimal Edge Detector". *International Journal of Computer Vision*, Vol. 1, No. 2, pp. 167–187, June 1987.

[Deri 90]   R. Deriche. "Fast Algorithms for Low-Level Vision". *IEEE Transactions on Pattern Analysis and Machine Intelligence*, Vol. 12, No. 1, pp. 78–87, January 1990.

[Deri 93]   R. Deriche. "Recursively Implementing the Gaussian and its Derivatives". Tech. Rep. 1893, Institute National de Recherche en Informatique et en Automatique (INRIA), April 1993.

[Desb 07]   L. Desbat, S. Roux, and P. Grangeat. "Compensation of some time dependent deformations in tomography". *IEEE Transactions on Medical Imaging*, Vol. 26, No. 2, pp. 261–269, February 2007.

[Desj 04]   B. Desjardins and E. A. Kazerooni. "ECG-gated Cardiac CT". *American Journal of Roentgenology*, Vol. 182, No. 4, pp. 993–1010, April 2004.

[Di C 06]   M. F. Di Carli and R. Hachamovitch. "Should PET replace SPECT for evaluating CAD? The end of the beginning". *Journal of Nuclear Cardiology*, Vol. 13, No. 1, pp. 2–7, January 2006.

[Di C 07a] M. F. Di Carli and S. Dorbala. *Myocardial Perfusion Imaging with PET*, In: M. F. Di Carli and M. J. Lipton, Eds., *Cardiac PET and PET/CT Imaging*, Chap. 11, pp. 151–159. Springer Verlag New York, xviii Ed., 2007.

[Di C 07b] M. F. Di Carli, S. Dorbala, J. Meserve, G. El Fakhri, A. Sitek, and S. C. Moore. "Clinical Myocardial Perfusion PET/CT". *The Journal of Nuclear Medicine*, Vol. 48, No. 5, pp. 783–793, May 2007.

[Dono 06]   D. L. Donoho. "Compressed Sensing". *IEEE Transactions on Information Theory*, Vol. 54, No. 4, pp. 1249–1306, April 2006.

[Drin 13]   M. Döring, F. Braunschweig, C. Eitel, T. Gaspar, U. Wetzel, B. Nitsche, G. Hindricks, and C. Piorkowski. "Individually tailored left ventricular lead placement: lessons from multimodality integration between three-dimensional echocardiography and coronary sinus angiogram". *Europace*, Vol. 15, No. 5, pp. 718–727, May 2013.

[Dsse 99]   O. Dössel. *Bildgebende Verfahren in der Medizin*. Springer Verlag Berlin Heidelberg, 1999 Ed., 1999.

[Ecto 09]   J. Ector, S. De Buck, D. Nuyens, T. Rossenbacker, W. Huybrechts, R. Gopal, F. Maes, and H. Heidbüchel. "Adenosine-induced ventricular asystole or rapid ventricular pacing to enhance three-dimensional rotational imaging during cardiac ablation procedures". *Europace*, Vol. 11, No. 6, pp. 751–762, June 2009.

[Erbe 07]   R. Erbel, S. Möhlenkamp, G. Kerkhoff, T. Budde, and A. Schmermund. "Non-invasive screening for coronary artery disease calcium scoring". *Heart*, Vol. 93, No. 12, pp. 1620–1629, December 2007.

[Euro 12]   European Society of Cardiology. "2012 European Cardiovascular Disease Statistics". http://www.escardio.org, September 2012. accessed 23rd November 2013.

[Fahr 97]   R. Fahrig, A. J. Fox, S. Lownie, and D. W. Holdsworth. "Use of a C-arm system to generate true three-dimensional computed rotational angiograms: preliminary in vitro and in vivo results". *American Journal of Neuroradiology*, Vol. 18, No. 8, pp. 1507–1514, September 1997.

[Feld 84]   L. A. Feldkamp, L. C. Davis, and J. W. Kress. "Practical cone-beam algorithm". *Journal of the Optical Society of America A*, Vol. 1, No. 6, pp. 612–619, June 1984.

[Flet 70]   R. Fletcher. "A new approach to variable metric algorithms". *The Computer Journal*, Vol. 13, No. 3, pp. 317–322, August 1970.

[Floh 08]   T. G. Flohr, H. Bruder, K. Stierstorfer, M. Petersilka, B. Schmidt, and H. Mc Collough. "Image reconstruction and image quality evaluation for a dual source CT scanner". *Medical Physics*, Vol. 35, No. 12, pp. 5882–5897, December 2008.

[Form 13]   C. Forman, R. Grimm, J. Hutter, A. Maier, J. Hornegger, and M. Zenge. "Free-Breathing Whole-Heart Coronary MRA: Motion Compensation Integrated into 3D Cartesian Compressed Sensing Reconstruction". In: K. Mori, I. Sakuma, Y. Sato, C. Barillot, and N. Navab, Eds., *Proceedings of the Medical Imaging and Computer Assisted Interventions (MICCAI) 2013*. Springer Verlag Berlin Heidelberg, *September 22-26, 2013, Nagoya, Japan.* pp. 575–582.

[Fort 08]   P. Forthmann, U. van Stevendaal, M. Grass, and T. Köhler. "Vector Field Interpolation for Cardiac Motion Compensated Reconstruction". In: *IEEE Nuclear Science Symposium Conference Record (NSS), 2008. October 19-25, 2008, Dresden, Germany.* pp. 4157–4160.

[Fran 01]   A. F. Frangi, W. J. Niessen, and M. A. Viergever. "Three-Dimensional Modeling for Functional Analysis of Cardiac Images: A Review". *IEEE Transactions on Medical Imaging*, Vol. 20, No. 1, pp. 2–25, January 2001.

[Gime 08]   V. M. Gimenes, M. L. Vieira, M. M. Andrade, J. Pinheiro Jr, V. T. Hotta, and W. Mathias Jr. "Standard Values for Real-Time Transthoracic Three-Dimensional Echocardiographic Dyssynchrony Indexes in a Normal Population". *Journal of the American Society of Echocardiography*, Vol. 21, No. 11, pp. 1229–1235, November 2008.

[Golu 96]   G. H. Golub and C. F. Van Loan. *Matrix Computations*. The Johns Hopkins University Press, 3rd Ed., 1996.

[Gord 70]   R. Gordon, R. Bender, and G. T. Herman. "Algebraic reconstruction techniques (ART) for three-dimensional electron microscopy and X-ray photography". *Journal of Theoretical Biology*, Vol. 29, No. 3, pp. 741–481, December 1970.

[Gran 02]   P. Grangeat, A. Koenig, T. Rodet, and S. Bonnet. "Theoretical framework for dynamic cone-beam reconstruction algorithm based on a dynamic particle model". *Physics in Medicine and Biology*, Vol. 47, No. 15, pp. 2611–2625, August 2002.

[Gran 91]   P. Grangeat. "Mathematical framework of cone beam 3D reconstruction via the first derivative of the radon transform". In: G. Herman, A. Louis, and F. Natterer, Eds., *Mathematical Methods in Tomography.* Springer Verlag Berlin Heidelberg, *June 5-11 1991, Oberwolfach, Germany.* pp. 66–97.

[Gray 00]   H. Gray. *Anatomy of the Human Body.* Twentieth Edition thoroughly revised and re-edited by Warren H. Lewis illustrated with 1247 Engravings Philadelphia: Lea and Febiger, 1918 New York, 20th Ed., 2000.

[Gupt 06]   R. Gupta, M. Grasruck, C. Suess, S. H. Bartling, B. Schmidt, K. Stierstorfer, S. Popescu, T. Brady, and T. Flohr. "Ultra-high resolution flat-panel volume CT: fundamental principles, design architecture, and system characterization". *European Radiology*, Vol. 16, No. 6, pp. 1191–1205, March 2006.

[Guru 08]   S. V. Gurudevan and J. Narula. "Prospective electrocardiogram-gating: a new direction for CT coronary angiography?". *Nature Clinical Practice Cardiovascular Medicine*, Vol. 5, No. 7, pp. 366–367, March 2008.

[Gutb 13]   M. Gutberlet. "Kardiale Magnetresonanztomographie". *Radiologe*, Vol. 53, No. 11, pp. 1033–1052, November 2013.

[Hahn 09] D. Hahn. *Statistical Medical Image Registration with Applications in Epilepsy Diagnosis and Shape-Based Segmentation*. PhD thesis, Universität Erlangen Nürnberg, 2009.

[Hans 08a] E. Hansis, D. Schäfer, O. Dössel, and M. Grass. "Evaluation of Iterative Sparse Object Reconstruction From Few Projections for 3-D Rotational Coronary Angiography". *IEEE Transactions on Medical Imaging*, Vol. 27, No. 11, pp. 1548–1555, October 2008.

[Hans 08b] E. Hansis, D. Schäfer, O. Dössel, and M. Grass. "Projection-based motion compensation for gated coronary artery reconstruction from rotational x-ray angiograms". *Physics in Medicine and Biology*, Vol. 53, No. 14, pp. 3807–3820, July 2008.

[Hans 09] E. Hansis, H. Schomberg, E. Klaus, O. Dössel, and M. Grass. "Four-dimensional cardiac reconstruction from rotational x-ray sequences: first results for 4D coronary angiography". In: E. Samei and J. Hsieh, Eds., *Proceedings of SPIE Medical Imaging 2009: Physics of Medical Imaging. February 7-12, 2009, Lake Buena Vista, FL, USA*. p. 72580B.

[Hart 04] R. Hartley and A. Zisserman. *Multiple View Geometry in Computer Vision*. Cambridge University Press, 2nd Ed., 2004.

[Herz 05] S. L. Herz, C. M. Ingrassia, S. Homma, K. D. Costa, and J. W. Holmes. "Parameterization of Left Ventricular Wall Motion for Detection of Regional Ischemia". *Annals of Biomedical Engineering*, Vol. 33, No. 7, pp. 912–919, July 2005.

[Hett 10] H. Hetterich, T. Redel, G. Lauritsch, C. Rohkohl, and J. Rieber. "New X-ray imaging modalities and their integration with intravascular imaging and interventions". *International Journal of Cardiovascular Imaging*, Vol. 26, No. 7, pp. 797–808, October 2010.

[Hija 09] Z. Hijazi, K. Shivkumar, and D. J. Sahn. "Intracardiac Echocardiography (ICE) During Interventional & Electrophysiological Cardiac Catheterization". *Circulation*, Vol. 119, No. 4, pp. 587–596, February 2009.

[Hoff 03] U. Hoffmann, T. J. Brady, and J. Muller. "Use of New Imaging Techniques to Screen for Coronary Artery Disease". *Circulation*, Vol. 108, pp. 50–53, August 2003.

[Hung 07] J. Hung, R. Lang, F. Flachskampf, S. K. Shernan, M. L. McCulloch, D. B. Adams, J. Thomas, M. Vannan, and T. Ryan. "3D Echocardiography: A Review of the Current Status and Future Directions". *Journal of the American Society of Echocardiography*, Vol. 20, No. 3, pp. 213–233, March 2007.

[Hunt 88] P. J. Hunter and B. H. Smaill. "The analysis of cardiac function: A continuum approach". *Progress In Biophysics and Molecular Biology*, Vol. 52, No. 2, pp. 101–164, 1988.

[Husm 07] L. Husmann, S. Leschka, L. Desbiolles, T. Schepis, O. Gaemperli, B. Seifert, P. Cattin, T. Frauenfelder, T. G. Flohr, B. Marincek, P. A. Kaufmann, and H. Alkadhi. "Coronary Artery Motion and Cardiac Phases: Dependency on Heart Rate Implications for CT Image Reconstruction". *Radiology*, Vol. 245, No. 2, pp. 567–576, November 2007.

[Isol 10a]   A. A. Isola, M. Grass, and W. J. Niessen. "Fully automatic nonrigid registration-based local motion estimation for motion-corrected iterative cardiac CT reconstruction". *Medical Physics*, Vol. 37, No. 3, pp. 1093–1109, March 2010.

[Isol 10b]   A. A. Isola, C. T. Metz, M. Schaap, S. Klein, W. J. Niessen, and M. Grass. "Coronary segmentation based motion corrected cardiac CT reconstruction". In: *IEEE Nuclear Science Symposium Conference Record Record (NSS/MIC), 2010. October 30 - November 6, 2010, Knoxville, TN, USA.* pp. 2026–2029.

[Isol 12]   A. Isola, C. Metz, M. Schaap, S. Klein, M. Grass, and W. Niessen. "Cardiac motion-corrected iterative cone-beam CT reconstruction using a semi-automatic minimum cost path-based coronary centerline extraction". *Medical Image Analysis*, Vol. 36, No. 3, pp. 215–226, April 2012.

[Jain 09]   A. Jain, L. Gutierrez, and D. Stanton. "3D TEE Registration with X-Ray Fluoroscopy for Interventional Cardiac Applications". In: N. Ayache, H. Delingette, and M. Sermesant, Eds., *Functional Imaging and Modeling of the Heart (FIMH) 2009. June 3-5, 2009, Nice, France.* pp. 321–329.

[Jenk 04]   C. Jenkins, K. Bricknell, L. Hanekom, and T. H. Marwick. "Reproducibility and accuracy of echocardiographic measurements of left ventricular parameters using real-time three-dimensional echocardiography". *Journal of the American College of Cardiology*, Vol. 44, No. 4, pp. 8788–886, August 2004.

[John 10]   M. John, R. Liao, Y. Zheng, A. Nöttling, J. Boese, U. Kirschstein, J. Kempfert, and T. Walther. "System to guide transcatheter aortic valve implantations based on interventional C-arm CT imaging". In: T. Jiang, N. Navab, J. Pluim, and M. Viergever, Eds., *Proceedings of the Medical Imaging and Computer Assisted Interventions (MICCAI) 2010.* Springer Verlag Berlin Heidelberg, *September 14-20, 2010, Beijing, China.* pp. 375–382.

[Jose 82]   P. M. Joseph. "An Improved Algorithm for Reprojecting Rays through Pixel Images". *IEEE Transactions on Medical Imaging*, Vol. 1, No. 3, pp. 192–196, November 1982.

[Kahn 12]   T. Kahn and H. Busse, Eds. *Interventional Magnetic Resonance Imaging. Medical Radiology*, Springer Verlag Berlin Heidelberg, xvii Ed., 2012.

[Kak 99]   A. C. Kak and M. Slaney. *Principles of Computerized Tomographic Imaging.* IEEE Press, 1999.

[Kale 08]   W. A. Kalender. "Technologische Entwicklungen in der MSCT". *Fortschritte auf dem Gebiet der Röntgenstrahlen und der Neuen Bildgebenden Verfahren - 87. Deutscher Röntgenkongress Supplement zum 87. Deutschen Röntgenkongress der DRG*, Vol. 178, No. S1, p. RK 221 1, May 2008.

[Kape 05]   S. Kapetanakis, M. T. Kearney, A. Siva, N. Gall, M. Cooklin, and M. J. Monaghan. "Real-Time Three-Dimensional Echocardiography A Novel Technique to Quantify Global Left Ventricular Mechanical Dyssynchrony". *Circulation*, Vol. 112, No. 7, pp. 992–1000, August 2005.

[Kats 03]   A. Katsevich. "A general scheme for constructing inversion algorithms for cone beam CT". *International Journal of Mathematics and Mathematical Sciences*, Vol. 2003, No. 21, pp. 1305–1321, September 2003.

[Kitz 90]   D. W. Kitzman and W. D. Edwards. "Age-Related Changes in the Anatomy of the Normal Human Heart". *The Journal of Gerontology*, Vol. 45, No. 2, pp. 33–39, 1990.

[Klei 09]   S. Klein, J. P. Pluim, M. Staring, and M. A. Viergever. "Adaptive Stochastic Gradient Descent Optimisation for Image Registration". *International Journal of Computer Vision*, Vol. 81, No. 3, pp. 227–239, March 2009.

[Klei 10]   S. Klein, M. Staring, K. Murphy, M. A. Viergever, and J. P. Pluim. "elastix: a toolbox for intensity based medical image registration". *IEEE Transactions on Medical Imaging*, Vol. 29, No. 1, pp. 196–205, January 2010.

[Knut 98]   D. Knuth. *Seminumerical Algorithms*. Vol. 2 of *The Art of Computer Programming*, Addison-Wesley Longman, 1998.

[Krak 04]   I. Krakau and H. Lapp. *Das Herzkatheterbuch Diagnostische und interventionelle Kathetertechniken*. Georg Thieme Verlag, 2nd Ed., 2004. p. 38/75.

[Kuwe 06]   T. Kuwert. "SPECT-CT versus PET-CT". http://www.european-hospital.com, July 2006. accessed 16/12/2013.

[Lang 12]   H. Langet, C. Riddell, Y. Trousset, A. Tenenhaus, E. Lahalle, G. Fleury, and N. Paragios. "Compressed sensing dynamic reconstruction in rotational angiography". In: N. Ayache, H. Delingette, P. Golland, and K. Mori, Eds., *Proceedings of the Medical Imaging and Computer Assisted Interventions (MICCAI) 2012*. Springer Verlag Berlin Heidelberg, *October 1-5, 2012, Nice, France*. pp. 223–230.

[Laur 06]   G. Lauritsch, J. Boese, L. Wigström, H. Kemeth, and R. Fahrig. "Towards Cardiac C-arm Computed Tomography". *IEEE Transactions on Medical Imaging*, Vol. 25, No. 7, pp. 922–934, July 2006.

[Lede 06]   R. J. Lederman. "Cardiovascular Interventional MRI". *Circulation*, Vol. 112, No. 19, pp. 3009–3017, November 2006.

[Lee 12]   H. Lee, S. Y. Kim, E. L. Hanna, and U. J. Schoepf. "Impact of ventricular contrast medium attenuation on the accuracy of left and right ventricular function analysis at cardiac multi detector-row CT compared with cardiac MRI". *Academic Radiology*, Vol. 19, No. 4, pp. 395–405, April 2012.

[Lewi 92]   R. M. Lewitt. "Alternatives to voxels for image representation in iterative reconstruction algorithms". *Physics in Medicine and Biology*, Vol. 37, No. 3, pp. 705–716, March 1992.

[Lust 07]   M. Lustig, D. Donoho, and J. M. Paly. "Sparse MRI: The Application of Compressed Sensing for Rapid MR Imaging". *Magnetic Resonance in Medicine*, Vol. 58, No. 6, pp. 1182–1195, 2007.

[Ma 12]   Y. L. Ma, A. K. Shetty, S. Duckett, P. Etyngier, G. Gijsbers, R. Bullens, T. Schaeffter, R. Razavi, C. A. Rinaldi, and K. S. Rhode. "An integrated platform for image-guided cardiac resynchronization therapy". *Physics in Medicine and Biology*, Vol. 57, No. 10, pp. 2953–2968, May 2012.

[Mahr 08]   H. Mahrholdt and U. Sechtem. "Gewebedifferenzierung mittels Kontrast-MRT ("late enhancement")". *Der Kardiologe*, Vol. 2, No. 3, pp. 215–226, June 2008.

[Maie 12]   A. Maier, H. Hofmann, C. Schwemmer, J. Hornegger, A. Keil, and R. Fahrig. "Fast simulation of X-ray projections of spline-based surfaces using an append buffer". *Physics in Medicine and Biology*, Vol. 57, No. 19, pp. 6193–6210, October 2012.

[Maie 13]   A. Maier, H. Hofmann, M. Berger, P. Fischer, C. Schwemmer, H. Wu, K. Müller, J. Hornegger, J.-H. Choi, C. Riess, A. Keil, and R. Fahrig. "CONRAD - A software framework for cone-beam imaging in radiology". *Medical Physics*, Vol. 40, No. 11, pp. 111914–1–8, November 2013.

[Mang 05]   N. E. Manghat, G. J. Morgan-Hughes, A. J. Marshall, and C. A. Roobottom. "Multidetector row computed tomography: imaging congenital coronary artery anomalies in adults". *Heart and Education in Heart*, Vol. 91, No. 12, pp. 1515–1522, December 2005.

[Manh 13]   M. T. Manhart, M. Kowarschik, A. Fieselmann, Y. Deuerling-Zheng, K. Royalty, A. Maier, and J. Hornegger. "Dynamic Iterative Reconstruction for Interventional 4-D C-Arm CT Perfusion Imaging". *IEEE Transactions on Medical Imaging*, Vol. 32, No. 7, pp. 2131–2138, July 2013.

[Mank 02]   D. Manke, K. Nehrke, P. Börnert, and O. Dössel. "Respiratory Motion in Coronary Magnetic Resonance Angiography: A Comparison of Different Motion Models". *Journal of Magnetic Resonance Imaging*, Vol. 15, No. 6, pp. 661–671, June 2002.

[Mant 08]   J. Mantilla, A. Bravo, and R. Medina. "A 3-D Multi-Modality Image Framework for Left Ventricle Motion Analysis". In: *International Machine Vision and Image Processing Conference (IMVIP). September 3-5, 2008, Portrush, UK.* pp. 130–135.

[Maro 06]   B. J. Maron and A. Pelliccia. "The Heart of Trained Athletes Cardiac Remodeling and the Risks of Sports, Including Sudden Death". *Circulation*, Vol. 114, No. 15, pp. 1633–1644, October 2006.

[Mate 96]   S. Matej and R. M. Lewitt. "Practical considerations for 3-D image reconstruction using spherically symmetric volume elements". *IEEE Transactions on Medical Imaging*, Vol. 15, No. 1, pp. 68–78, February 1996.

[Matt 12]   S. Matthew, S. Gandy, R. Nicholas, S. Waugh, E. Crowe, R. Lerski, M. Dunn, and J. Houston. "Quantitative analysis of cardiac left ventricular variables obtained by MRI at 3 T: a pre- and post-contrast comparison". *British Journal of Radiology*, Vol. 85, No. 1015, pp. 343–347, July 2012.

[Medi 06]   R. Medina, M. Garreau, J. Toro, H. L. Breton, J. L. Coatrieux, and D. Jugo. "Markov Random Field Modeling for Three-Dimensional Reconstruction of the Left Ventricle in Cardiac Angiography". *IEEE Transactions on Medical Imaging*, Vol. 25, No. 8, pp. 1087–1100, August 2006.

[Metz 13]   C. T. Metz, M. Schaap, S. Klein, N. Baka, L. A. Neefjes, C. J. Schultz, W. J. Niessen, and T. van Walsum. "Registration of 3D+t coronary CTA and monoplane 2D+t X-ray angiography". *IEEE Transactions on Medical Imaging*, Vol. 32, No. 5, pp. 919–931, May 2013.

[Mkel 02]   T. Mäkelä, P. Clarysse, O. Sipilä, N. Pauna, Q. C. Pham, and I. E. Katila, T. Magning. "A Review of Cardiac Image Registration Methods". *IEEE Transactions on Medical Imaging*, Vol. 21, No. 9, pp. 1011–1021, 2002.

[Mlle 12a]   K. Müller, C. Rohkohl, G. Lauritsch, C. Schwemmer, H. Heidbüchel, S. De Buck, D. Nuyens, Y. Kyriakou, C. Köhler, and J. Hornegger. "4-D Motion Field Estimation by Combined Multiple Heart Phase Registration (CMHPR) for Cardiac C-arm Data". In: *IEEE Nuclear Science Symposium and Medical Imaging Conference Record (NSS/MIC), 2012. October 27 - November 3, 2012, Anaheim, CA, USA*. pp. 3707–3712.

[Mlle 12b]   K. Müller, Y. Zheng, G. Lauritsch, C. Rohkohl, C. Schwemmer, A. Maier, R. Fahrig, and J. Hornegger. "Evaluation of Interpolation Methods for Motion Compensated Tomographic Reconstruction for Cardiac Angiographic C-arm Data". In: F. Noo, Ed., *Proceedings of The Second International Conference on Image Formation in X-Ray Computed Tomography. June 24-27, 2012, Salt Lake City, UT, USA*. pp. 5–8.

[Mlle 13a]   K. Müller, G. Lauritsch, C. Schwemmer, and C. Rohkohl. "Kombinierte, multiple Herzphasenregistrierung in der kardialen Bildrekonstruktion für den Angio C-Bogen". 2013. Patent No. 13/959,011.

[Mlle 13b]   K. Müller, A. Maier, P. Fischer, B. Bier, G. Lauritsch, C. Schwemmer, R. Fahrig, and J. Hornegger. "Left Ventricular Heart Phantom for Wall Motion Analysis". In: *IEEE Nuclear Science Symposium and Medical Imaging Conference Record (NSS/MIC), 2013. October 27 - November 2, 2013, Seoul, Korea*.

[Mlle 13c]   K. Müller, C. Schwemmer, J. Hornegger, Y. Zheng, Y. Wang, G. Lauritsch, A. Maier, C. Schultz, and R. Fahrig. "Evaluation of interpolation methods for surface-based motion compensated tomographic reconstruction for cardiac angiographic C-arm data". *Medical Physics*, Vol. 40, No. 3, pp. 031107–1 –12, February 2013.

[Mlle 13d]   K. Müller, C. Schwemmer, G. Lauritsch, C. Rohkohl, A. Maier, H. Heidbüchel, S. De Buck, D. Nuyens, Y. Kyriakou, C. Köhler, R. Fahrig, and J. Hornegger. "Image Artifact Influence on Motion Compensated Tomographic Reconstruction in Cardiac C-arm CT". In: R. Leahy and J. Qi, Eds., *Proceedings of the 12th International Meeting on Fully Three-Dimensional Image Reconstruction in Radiology and Nuclear Medicine (Fully3D). June 16-21, 2013, Lake Tahoe, CA, USA*. pp. 98–101.

[Mlle 14a]   K. Müller, G. Lauritsch, C. Schwemmer, A. K. Maier, B. Abt, H. Köhler, A. Nöttling, J. Hornegger, and R. Fahrig. "Catheter Artifact Reduction (CAR) in Dynamic Cardiac Chamber Imaging with Interventional C-arm CT". In: F. Noo, Ed., *Proceedings of The Third International Conference on Image Formation in X-Ray Computed Tomography. June 22-25, 2014, Salt Lake City, UT, USA*. p. accepted for publication.

[Mlle 14b]   K. Müller, A. Maier, C. Schwemmer, G. Lauritsch, S. De Buck, J.-Y. Wielandts, J. Hornegger, and R. Fahrig. "Image Artefact Propagation in Motion Estimation and Reconstruction in Interventional Cardiac C-arm

CT". *Physics in Medicine and Biology*, Vol. 59, No. 12, pp. 3097–3119, May 2014.

[Mlle 14c]   K. Müller, A. Maier, Y. Zheng, Y. Wang, G. Lauritsch, C. Schwemmer, C. Rohkohl, J. Hornegger, and R. Fahrig. "Interventional Heart Wall Motion Analysis with Cardiac C-arm CT Systems". *Physics in Medicine and Biology*, Vol. 59, No. 9, pp. 2265–2284, April 2014.

[Mode 03]   J. Modersitzki. *Numerical Methods for Image Registration (Numerical Mathematics and Scientific Computation)*. Oxford University Press, 2003.

[Mori 02]   M. Moriyama, Y. Sato, H. Naito, M. Hanayama, T. Ueguchi, T. Harada, F. Yoshimoto, and S. Tamura. "Reconstruction of Time-Varying 3-D Left-Ventricular Shape From Multiview X-Ray Cineangiocardiograms". *IEEE Transactions on Medical Imaging*, Vol. 21, No. 7, pp. 773–785, July 2002.

[Mory 14]   C. Mory, V. Auvray, B. Zhang, M. Grass, D. Schäfer, S. J. Chen, J. D. Carroll, S. Rit, F. Peyrin, P. Douek, and L. Boussel. "Cardiac C-arm computed tomography using a 3D + time ROI reconstruction method with spatial and temporal regularization". *Medical Physics*, Vol. 41, No. 2, pp. 0219031–12, February 2014.

[Moyn 81]   P. F. Moynihan, A. F. Parisi, and C. L. Feldman. "Quantitative detection of regional left ventricular contraction abnormalities by two-dimensional echocardiography. I. Analysis of methods". *Circulation*, Vol. 63, No. 4, pp. 752–760, April 1981.

[Mura 10]   D. Muraru, L. Badano, G. Piccoli, P. Gianfagna, L. Del Mestre, D. Ermacora, and A. Proclemer. "Validation of a novel automated border-detection algorithm for rapid and accurate quantitation of left ventricular volumes based on three-dimensional echocardiography". *European Journal of Echocardiography*, Vol. 11, No. 4, pp. 359–368, May 2010.

[Nava 98]   N. Navab, A. Bani-Hashemi, M. Nadar, K. Wiesent, P. Durlak, T. Brunner, K. Barth, and R. Graumann. "3D reconstruction from projection matrices in a C-arm based 3D-angiography system". In: W. Wells, A. Colchester, and S. Delp, Eds., *Proceedings of the Medical Imaging and Computer Assisted Interventions (MICCAI) 1998*. Springer Verlag Berlin Heidelberg, *October 11-13, 1998, Cambridge, MA, USA*. pp. 119–129.

[Naza 13]   S. Nazarian, R. Beinart, and H. Halpein. "Magnetic Resonance Imaging and Implantable Devices". *Circulation*, Vol. 6, No. 2, pp. 419–428, April 2013.

[Nehr 01]   K. Nehrke, P. Börnert, D. Manke, and J. Böck. "Free-breathing Cardiac MR Imaging: Study of Implications of Respiratory Motion - Initial Results". *Radiology*, Vol. 220, No. 3, pp. 810–815, September 2001.

[Nett 08a]   B. Nett, J. Tang, S. Leng, and G.-H. Chen. "Tomosynthesis via Total Variation Minimization Reconstruction and Prior Image Constrained Compressed Sensing (PICCS) on a C-arm System". In: E. Samei and J. Hsieh, Eds., *Proceedings of SPIE Medical Imaging 2008: Physics of Medical Imaging*. *February 16-21, 2008, San Diego, CA, USA*. p. 69132D.

[Nett 08b] F. Netter. *Atlas der Anatomie des Menschen*. Elsevier Urban & Fischer München, 4th Ed., 2008.

[Newe 09] M. Newell, A. Doonan, J. Lesser, and R. Schwartz. "3-D Rotational Angiography in the Cardiac Cath Lab". *The Journal of Invasive Cardiology*, Vol. 21, No. 7, pp. 336–338, July 2009.

[Nlke 10] G. Nölker, S. Asbach, K. Gutleben, H. Rittger, G. Ritscher, J. Brachmann, and A. Sinha. "Image-integration of intraprocedural rotational angiography-based 3D reconstructions of left atrium and pulmonary veins into electroanatomical mapping: accuracy of a novel modality in atrial fibrillation ablation". *Journal of Cardiovascular Electrophysiology*, Vol. 21, No. 3, pp. 278–283, March 2010.

[Noo 07] F. Noo, S. Hoppe, F. Dennerlein, G. Lauritsch, and J. Hornegger. "A new scheme for view-dependent data differentiaton in fan-beam and cone-beam computed tomography". *Physics in Medicine and Biology*, Vol. 52, No. 17, pp. 5393–5414, August 2007.

[Noo 12] F. Noo, K. Schmitt, K. Stierstorfer, and H. Schöndube. "Image representation using mollified pixels for iterative reconstruction in X-ray CT". In: *IEEE Nuclear Science Symposium and Medical Imaging Conference Record (NSS/MIC), 2012. October 29 - November 2012, 2012, Anaheim, CA, USA*. pp. 3453–3455.

[Nyul 00] L. Nyul, J. Udupa, , and X. Zhang. "New Variants of a Method of MRI Scale Standardization". *IEEE Transactions on Medical Imaging*, Vol. 19, No. 2, pp. 143–150, February 2000.

[Orth 09] R. Orth, M. Wallace, and M. Kuo. "C-arm Cone-beam CT: General Principles and Technical Considerations for Use in Interventional Radiology". *Journal of Vascular and Interventional Radiology*, Vol. 19, No. 6, pp. 814–820, June 2009.

[Park 82] D. Parker. "Optimal short scan convolution reconstruction for fan beam CT". *Medical Physics*, Vol. 9, No. 2, pp. 254–257, March 1982.

[Penn 98] G. Penney, J. Weese, J. Little, P. Desmedt, D. Hill, and D. Hawkes. "A comparison of similarity measures for use in 2-D-3-D medical image registration". *IEEE Transactions on Medical Imaging*, Vol. 17, No. 4, pp. 586–595, August 1998.

[Penn 99] X. Pennec, P. Cachier, and N. Ayache. "Understanding the 'Demon's Algorithm': 3D Non-Rigid registration by Gradient Descent". In: C. Taylor and A. Colchester, Eds., *Proceedings of the Medical Imaging and Computer Assisted Interventions (MICCAI) 1999*. Springer Verlag Berlin Heidelberg, *September 19-22, 1999, Cambridge, UK*. pp. 597–605.

[Perp 05] D. Perperidis, R. Mohiaddin, and D. Rueckert. "Spatio-temporal free-form registration of cardiac MR image sequences". *Medical Image Analysis*, Vol. 9, No. 5, pp. 441–456, October 2005.

[Pfis 85] M. Pfisterer, A. Battler, and B. Zaret. "Range of normal values for left and right ventricular ejection fraction at rest and during exercise assessed by radionuclide angiocardiography". *European Heart Journal*, Vol. 6, No. 8, pp. 647–655, August 1985.

[Po 11]   M. Po, M. Srichai, and A. Laine. "Quantitative detection of left ven-
            tricular dyssynchrony from cardiac computed tomography angiography".
            In: *Proceedings of the 8th IEEE International Symposium on Biomedical
            Imaging: From Nano to Macro (ISBI 2011). March 30 - April 2, 2011,
            Chicago, IL, USA.* pp. 1318–1321.

[Prmm 06a] M. Prümmer, J. Hornegger, M. Pfister, and A. Dörfler. "Multi-modal
            2D-3D Non-rigid Registration". In: J. Reinhardt and J. Pluim, Eds.,
            *Proceedings of SPIE Medical Imaging 2006: Image Processing. February
            2006, San Diego, CA, USA.* p. 61440X.

[Prmm 06b] M. Prümmer, L. Wigström, J. Hornegger, J. Boese, G. Lauritsch,
            N. Strobel, and R. Fahrig. "Cardiac C-arm CT: Efficient Motion Cor-
            rection for 4D-FBP". In: *IEEE Nuclear Science Symposium Conference
            Record (NSS), 2006. October 29 - November 1, 2006, San Diego, CA,
            USA.* pp. 2620–2628.

[Prmm 09a] M. Prümmer. *Cardiac C-Arm Computed Tomography: Motion Esti-
            mation and Dynamic Reconstruction.* PhD thesis, Friedrich-Alexander-
            Universität Erlangen-Nürnberg, 2009.

[Prmm 09b] M. Prümmer, J. Hornegger, G. Lauritsch, L. Wigström, E. Girard-
            Hughes, and R. Fahrig. "Cardiac C-Arm CT: A Unified Framework for
            Motion Estimation and Dynamic CT". *IEEE Transactions on Medical
            Imaging*, Vol. 28, No. 11, pp. 1836–1849, November 2009.

[Qian 10]   Z. Qian, H. Anderson, I. Marvasty, K. Akram, G. Vazquez, S. Rinehart,
            and S. Voros. "Lesion- and vessel-specific coronary artery calcium scores
            are superior to whole-heart Agatston and volume scores in the diagno-
            sis of obstructive coronary artery disease". *Journal of Cardiovascular
            Computed Tomography*, Vol. 4, No. 6, pp. 391–399, November 2010.

[Rahm 08]   A. Rahmim and H. Zaidi. "PET versus SPECT: strengths, limitations
            and challenges". *Nuclear Medicine Communications*, Vol. 29, No. 3,
            pp. 193–207, March 2008.

[Rami 11]   J. C. Ramirez-Giraldo, J. Trzasko, S. Leng, L. Yu, A. Manduca, and
            C. H. McCollough. "Nonconvex prior image constrained compressed
            sensing (NCPICCS): Theory and simulations on perfusion CT". *Medical
            Physics*, Vol. 38, No. 4, pp. 2157–2167, April 2011.

[Rcke 99]   D. Rückert, L. I. Sonoda, C. Hayes, D. L. Hill, M. O. Leach, and
            D. Hawkes. "Nonrigid registration using free-form deformations: Appli-
            cation to breast MR images". *IEEE Transactions on Medical Imaging*,
            Vol. 18, No. 8, pp. 712–721, August 1999.

[Rieb 09]   J. Rieber, C. Rohkohl, G. Lauritsch, H. Rittger, and O. Meissner. "Kar-
            diale Anwendung der C-Arm-Computertomographie". *Der Radiologe*,
            Vol. 49, No. 9, pp. 862–867, September 2009.

[Rits 10]   L. Ritschl, F. Bergner, C. Fleischmann, and M. Kachelrieß. "Improved
            sparsity-constrained image reconstruction applied to clinical CT data".
            In: *IEEE Nuclear Science Symposium and Medical Imaging Conference
            Record (NSS/MIC), 2010. October 30 - November 6, 2010, Knoxville,
            TN, USA.* pp. 3231–3240.

[Rits 11]   L. Ritschl, F. Bergner, C. Fleischmann, and M. Kachelrieß. "Improved
              total variation-based CT image reconstruction applied to clinical data".
              Physics in Medicine and Biology, Vol. 56, No. 6, pp. 1545–1562, February
              2011.

[Robb 51]   H. Robbins and S. Monro. "A stochastic approximation method". *The
              Annals of Mathematical Statistics*, Vol. 22, No. 3, pp. 400–407, Septem-
              ber 1951.

[Rohk 08]   C. Rohkohl, G. Lauritsch, A. Nöttling, M. Prümmer, and J. Hornegger.
              "C-arm CT: Reconstruction of Dynamic High Contrast Objects Applied
              to the Coronary Sinus". In: *IEEE Nuclear Science Symposium Con-
              ference Record (NSS), 2008. Dresden, October 19-25, 2008, Dresden,
              Germany*. pp. 5113–5120.

[Rohk 10a]   C. Rohkohl. *Motion Estimation and Compensation for Interventional
              Cardiovascular Image Reconstruction*. PhD thesis, Friedrich-Alexander-
              Universität Erlangen-Nürnberg, 2010.

[Rohk 10b]   C. Rohkohl, G. Lauritsch, L. Biller, M. Prümmer, J. Boese, and
              J. Hornegger. "Interventional 4D motion estimation and reconstruction
              of cardiac vasculature without motion periodicity assumption". *Medical
              Image Analysis*, Vol. 14, No. 5, pp. 687–694, October 2010.

[Rohk 13]   C. Rohkohl, H. Bruder, K. Stierstorfer, and T. Flohr. "Improving best-
              phase image quality in cardiac CT by motion correction with MAM
              optimization". *Medical Physics*, Vol. 40, No. 3, pp. 031901-1–15, March
              2013.

[Rohr 01]   K. Rohr, H. S. Stiehl, R. Sprengel, T. M. Buzug, J. Weese, and M. H.
              Kuhn. "Landmark-Based Elastic Registration Using Approximating
              Thin-Plate Splines". *IEEE Transactions on Medical Imaging*, Vol. 20,
              No. 6, pp. 526–534, June 2001.

[Roth 11]   E. Rothgang, W. D. Gilson, W. Strehl, L. Pan, J. Roland, C. H. Lorenz,
              and J. Hornegger. "Interventional MR-Imaging for Thermal Ablation
              Therapy". In: *Proceedings of the 8th IEEE International Symposium on
              Biomedical Imaging: From Nano to Macro (ISBI 2011). March 30 -
              April 2, 2011, Chicago, IL, USA*. pp. 1864–1868.

[Roug 93]   A. Rougée, C. Picard, C. Ponchut, and Y. Trousset. "Geometrical cal-
              ibration of x-ray imaging chains for three-dimensional reconstruction".
              Computerized Medical Imaging and Graphics, Vol. 17, No. 4-5, pp. 295–
              300, October 1993.

[Russ 03]   D. B. Russakoff, T. Rohlfing, A. Ho, D. H. Kim, R. Shahidi, J. R.
              Adler Jr, and C. R. Maurer Jr. "Evaluation of Intensity-Based 2D-
              3D Spine Image Registration Using Clinical Gold-Standard Data". In:
              J. Gee, J. Maintz, and M. Vannier, Eds., *Biomedical Image Registration*,
              pp. 151–160, Springer Verlag Berlin Heidelberg, 2003.

[Sach 11]   V. Sachpekidis, A. Bhan, and M. J. Monaghan. *Three-dimensional
              Echocardiography Evaluation of LV Dyssynchrony and Stress Testing*,
              In: L. Badano, R. M. Lang, and J. L. Zamorano, Eds., *Textbook of Real-
              Time Three Dimensional Echocardiography*, Chap. 7, pp. 64–67. Springer
              Verlag London Limited, xii Ed., 2011.

[Sain 94]   D. Saint-Félix, Y. Trousset, C. Picard, C. Ponchut, R. Roméas, and
             A. Rougée. "In vivo evaluation of a new system for 3D computerized
             angiography". *Physics in Medicine and Biology*, Vol. 39, No. 3, pp. 583–
             595, March 1994.

[Sand 10]   J. Sanders and E. Kandrot. *CUDA by Example: An Introduction to
             General-Purpose GPU Programming*. Addison-Wesley Longman, Ams-
             terdam, 1st Ed., 2010.

[Sche 11]   H. Scherl. *Evaluation of State-of-the-Art Hardware Architectures for
             Fast Cone-Beam CT Reconstruction*. PhD thesis, Friedrich-Alexander-
             Universität Erlangen-Nürnberg, 2011.

[Schf 06]   D. Schäfer, J. Borgert, V. Rasche, and M. Grass. "Motion-Compensated
             and Gated Cone Beam Filtered Back-Projection for 3-D Rotational X-
             Ray Angiography". *IEEE Transactions on Medical Imaging*, Vol. 25,
             No. 7, pp. 898–906, July 2006.

[Schi 10]   T. H. Schindler, H. R. Schelbert, A. Quercioli, and V. Dilsizian. "Car-
             diac PET Imaging for the Detection and Monitoring of Coronary Artery
             Disease and Microvascular Health". *Journal of the American College of
             Cardiology*, Vol. 3, No. 6, pp. 623–640, June 2010.

[Schm 12]   K. Schmitt, F. Noo, J. Hornegger, K. Stierstorfer, and H. Schöndube. "It-
             erative reconstruction using a pyramid-shaped basis function". In: *IEEE
             Nuclear Science Symposium and Medical Imaging Conference Record
             (NSS/MIC), 2012. October 27 - November 3, 2012, Anaheim, CA, USA*.
             pp. 3456–3460.

[Schn 11]   H. Schöndube, T. Allmendinger, K. Stierstorfer, H. Bruder, and T. Flohr.
             "Evaluation of a novel CT image reconstruction algorithm with enhanced
             temporal resolution". In: N. Pelc, E. Samei, and R. Nishikawa, Eds.,
             *Proceedings of SPIE Medical Imaging 2011: Physics of Medical Imaging.
             February 12-17, 2011, Lake Buena Vista, FL, USA*. p. 79611N.

[Scho 07]   H. Schomberg. "Time-Resolved Cardiac Cone Beam CT". In: M. Kachel-
             riess, F. Beekmann, and K. Müller, Eds., *Proceedings of the 9th Inter-
             national Meeting on Fully Three-Dimensional Image Reconstruction in
             Radiology and Nuclear Medicine (Fully3D). July 9-13, 2007, Lindau,
             Germany*. pp. 362–365.

[Schr 06]   W. Schroeder, K. Martin, and B. Lorensen. *The Visualization Toolkit:
             An Object-Oriented Approach To 3D Graphics*. Kitware, Inc., 4 Ed.,
             2006.

[Schr 09]   J. Schrader, A. Gödecke, and M. Kelm. *Physiologie*. Thieme Verlag,
             Stuttgart, 6 Ed., November 2009.

[Schu 13]   C. J. Schultz, N. M. van Mieghem, R. M. van der Boon, A. S. Dharampal,
             G. Lauritsch, A. Rossi, A. Moelker, G. Krestin, R. van Geuns, P. de Fei-
             jter, P. W. Serruys, and P. de Jaegere. "Effect of body mass index on
             the image quality of rotational angiography without rapid pacing for
             planning of transcatheter aortic valve implantation: a comparison with
             multislice computed tomography". *European Heart Journal Cardiovas-
             cular Imaging*, Vol. 15, No. 2, pp. 133–141, March 2013.

[Schw 10]   C. Schwemmer, M. Prümmer, V. Daum, and J. Hornegger. "High-Density Object Removal from Projection Images using Low-Frequency-Based Object Masking". In: T. Deserno, H. Handels, H.-P. Meinzer, and T. Tolxdorf, Eds., *Bildverarbeitung für die Medizin 2010 - Algorithmen - Systeme - Anwendungen*. Springer Verlag Berlin Heidelberg, *March 14-16 2010, Aachen*. pp. 365–369.

[Schw 11]   J. G. Schwartz, A. M. Neubauer, T. E. Fagan, N. J. Noordhoek, M. Grass, and J. D. Carroll. "Potential role of three-dimensional rotational angiography and C-arm CT for valvular repair and implantation". *International Journal of Cardiovascular Imaging*, Vol. 27, No. 8, pp. 1205–1222, December 2011.

[Schw 13]   C. Schwemmer, C. Rohkohl, G. Lauritsch, K. Müller, and J. Hornegger. "Residual Motion Compensation in ECG-Gated Interventional Cardiac Vasculature Reconstruction". *Physics in Medicine and Biology*, Vol. 58, No. 11, pp. 3717–3737, June 2013.

[Sega 08]   W. P. Segars, M. Mahesh, T. J. Beck, E. C. Frey, and B. M. W. Tsui. "Realistic CT simulation using the 4D XCAT phantom". *Medical Physics*, Vol. 35, No. 8, pp. 3800–3808, August 2008.

[Sega 99]   W. P. Segars, D. S. Lalush, and B. M. W. Tsui. "A realistic spline-based dynamic heart phantom". *IEEE Transactions on Nuclear Science*, Vol. 46, No. 3, pp. 503–506, June 1999.

[Shaw 14]   C. C. Shaw, Ed. *Cone Beam Computed Tomography (Imaging in Medical Diagnosis and Therapy)*. Taylor and Francis, 1st Ed., 2014.

[Shec 03]   G. Shechter, F. Devernay, E. Coste-Maniére, A. Quyyumi, and E. R. Mc Veigh. "Three-dimensional motion tracking of coronary arteries in biplane cineangiograms". *IEEE Transactions on Medical Imaging*, Vol. 22, No. 4, pp. 493–503, April 2003.

[Shep 68]   D. Shepard. "A two-dimensional interpolation function for irregularly-spaced data". In: R. Blue and A. Rosenberg, Eds., *ACM '68 Proceedings of the 1968 23rd ACM national conference. August 27-29, 1968, Las Vegas, NV, USA*. pp. 517–524.

[Shep 82]   L. A. Shepp and B. Logan. "Reconstructing Interior Head Tissue From X-ray Transmissions". *IEEE Transactions on Nuclear Science*, Vol. 1, No. 2, pp. 228–236, February 1982.

[Sidd 85]   R. L. Siddon. "Fast calculation of the exact radiological path for a threedimensional CT array". *Medical Physics*, Vol. 12, No. 2, pp. 252–255, April 1985.

[Sidk 06]   E. Y. Sidky, C.-M. Kao, and X. Pan. "Accurate image reconstruction from few-views and limited-angle data in divergent-beam CT". *Journal of X-Ray Science and Technology*, Vol. 14, No. 2, pp. 119–139, June 2006.

[Sidk 08]   E. Y. Sidky and X. Pan. "Image reconstruction in circular cone-beam computed tomography by constrained, total-variation minimization". *Physics in Medicine and Biology*, Vol. 53, No. 17, pp. 4777–4807, August 2008.

[Soti 13]   A. Sotiras, C. Davatzikos, and N. Paragios. "Deformable Medical Image Registration: A Survey". *IEEE Transactions on Medical Imaging*, Vol. 32, No. 7, pp. 1153–1190, May 2013.

[Spre 96]   R. Sprengel, K. Rohr, and H. S. Stiehl. "Thin-plate spline approximation for image registration". In: *Proceedings of the 18th Annual International Conference of the IEEE Engineering in Medicine and Biology Society, 1996. Bridging Disciplines for Biomedicine. October 31 - November 3, 1996, Amsterdam, The Netherlands*. pp. 1190–1191.

[Stro 09]   N. Strobel, O. Meissner, J. Boese, T. Brunner, B. Heigl, M. Hoheisel, G. Lauritsch, M. Nagel, M. Pfister, E. P. Rührnschopf, B. Scholz, B. Schreiber, M. Spahn, M. Zellerhoff, and K. Klingenbeck-Regn. *Imaging with Flat-Detector C-Arm Systems*, In: M. F. Reiser, C. R. Becker, K. Nikolaou, and G. Glazer, Eds., *Multislice CT (Medical Radiology / Diagnostic Imaging)*, Chap. 3, pp. 33–51. Springer Verlag Berlin Heidelberg, 3rd Ed., 2009.

[Stru 09]   T. Struffert and A. Doerfler. "Flachdetektor-CT in der diagnostischen und interventionellen Neuroradiologie". *Der Radiologe*, Vol. 49, No. 9, pp. 820–829, September 2009.

[Sute 00]   D. Suter and F. Chen. "Left Ventricular Motion Reconstruction Based on Elastic Vector Splines". *IEEE Transactions on Medical Imaging*, Vol. 19, No. 4, pp. 295–305, April 2000.

[Swob 05]   R. Swoboda, M. Carpella, C. Steinwender, C. Gabriel, F. Leisch, and W. Backfrieder. "From 2D to 4D in Quantitative Left Ventricle Wall Motion Analysis of Biplanar X-Ray Angiograms". In: *Computers in Cardiology. September 25-28 2005, Lyon, FR*. pp. 977–980.

[Tagu 07]   K. Taguchi and H. Kudo. "Motion compensated fan-beam reconstruction for computed tomography using derivative backprojection filtering approach". In: M. Kachelriess, F. Beekmann, and K. Müller, Eds., *Proceedings of the 9th International Meeting on Fully Three-Dimensional Image Reconstruction in Radiology and Nuclear Medicine (Fully3D). July 9-13, 2007, Lindau, Germany*. pp. 433–436.

[Tagu 08]   K. Taguchi and H. Kudo. "Motion Compensated Fan-Beam Reconstruction for Nonrigid Transformation". *IEEE Transactions on Medical Imaging*, Vol. 27, No. 7, pp. 907–917, July 2008.

[Tang 12]   Q. Tang, J. Cammin, S. Srivastava, and K. Taguchi. "A fully four-dimensional, iterative motion estimation and compensation method for cardiac CT". *Medical Physics*, Vol. 39, No. 7, pp. 4291–4305, July 2012.

[Tang 13]   J. Tang, J. Cammin, and K. Taguchi. "Four-dimensional projection-based motion estimation and compensation for cardiac x-ray computed tomography". In: R. Leahy and J. Qi, Eds., *Proceedings of the 12th International Meeting on Fully Three-Dimensional Image Reconstruction in Radiology and Nuclear Medicine (Fully3D). June 16-21, 2013, Lake Tahoe, CA, USA*. pp. 46–49.

[Thir 98]   J. P. Thirion. "Image matching as a diffusion process: an analogy with Maxwell's demons". *Medical Image Analysis*, Vol. 2, No. 3, pp. 243–260, September 1998.

[Thri 12a] P. Thèriault-Lauzier and G.-H. Chen. "Characterization of statistical prior image constrained compressed sensing. I. Applications to time-resolved contrast-enhanced CT". *Medical Physics*, Vol. 39, No. 10, pp. 5930–5948, October 2012.

[Thri 12b] P. Thèriault-Lauzier, J. Tang, and G. H. Chen. "Prior image constrained compressed sensing: Implementation and performance evaluation". *Medical Physics*, Vol. 39, No. 1, pp. 66–80, January 2012.

[Thri 12c] P. Thèriault-Lauzier, J. Tang, and G.-H. Chen. "Time-resolved cardiac interventional cone-beam CT reconstruction from fully truncated projections using the prior image constrained compressed sensing (PICCS) algorithm". *Physics in Medicine and Biology*, Vol. 57, No. 9, pp. 2461–2476, May 2012.

[Thri 13] P. Thèriault-Lauzier and G.-H. Chen. "Characterization of statistical prior image constrained compressed sensing. II. Application to dose reduction". *Medical Physics*, Vol. 40, No. 2, pp. 021902-1–14, February 2013.

[Toma 98] C. Tomasi. "Bilateral Filtering for Gray and Color Images". In: *Sixth International Conference on Computer Vision 1998. January 4-7, 1998, Bombay, India.* pp. 839–846.

[Tu 05] Z. Tu. "Probabilistic boosting-tree: learning discriminative models for classification, recognition, and clustering". In: *Tenth IEEE International Conference on Computer Vision, 2005 (ICCV 2005). October 17-20, 2005, Beijing, China.* pp. 1589–1596.

[Tuy 83] H. Tuy. "An Inversion Formula for Cone-Beam Reconstruction". *SIAM Journal on Applied Mathematics*, Vol. 43, No. 3, pp. 546–552, June 1983.

[Ulzh 09] S. Ulzheimer and T. Flohr. *Multislice CT: Current Technology and Future Developments*, In: M. F. Reiser, C. R. Becker, K. Noikolaou, and G. Glazer, Eds., *Multislice CT (Medical Radiology)*, Chap. Current Technology and Future Developments, pp. 3–23. Springer Verlag Berlin Heidelberg, 2009.

[Unse 99] M. Unser. "Splines: A perfect fit for signal and image processing". *IEEE Signal Processing Magazine*, Vol. 16, No. 6, pp. 22–38, November 1999.

[US D 12] U.S. Department of Health and Human Services. "Death: Preliminary Data for 2011". *National Vital Statistics and Reports (NVSS)*, Vol. 61, No. 6, pp. 1–52, October 2012.

[Verc 07] T. Vercauteren, X. Pennec, A. Perchant, and N. Ayache. "Diffeomorphic Demons Using ITK's Finite Difference Solver Hierarchy". In: N. Ayache, S. Ourselin, and A. J. Maeder, Eds., *The Insight Journal - 2007 MICCAI Open Science Workshop at MICCAI. October 29 - November 2, 2007, Brisbane, Australia.* pp. 1–8.

[Verc 09] T. Vercauteren, X. Pennec, A. Perchant, and N. Ayache. "Diffeomorphic demons: efficient non-parametric image registration". *NeuroImage*, Vol. 45, No. 1, pp. 61–72, March 2009.

[Vovk 07] U. Vovk, F. Pernus, and B. Likar. "A review of Methods for correction of intensity inhomogeniety in MRI". *IEEE Transactions on Medical Imaging*, Vol. 26, No. 3, pp. 405–421, March 2007.

[Wall 09]   M. J. Wallace, M. D. Kuo, C. Glaiberman, C. A. Binkert, R. C. Orth, and G. Soulez. "Three-Dimensional C-arm Cone-beam CT: Applications in the Interventional Suite". *Journal of Vascular and Interventional Radiology*, Vol. 20, No. 7, pp. 523–537, July 2009.

[Wang 02]   Z. Wang and A. C. Bovik. "A Universal Image Quality Index". *IEEE Signal Processing Letters*, Vol. 9, No. 3, pp. 81–84, March 2002.

[Wang 05]   H. Wang, L. Dong, J. O'Daniel, R. Mohan, A. S. Garden, K. K. Ang, D. A. Kuban, M. Bonnen, J. Y. Chang, and R. Cheung. "Validation of an accelerated 'demons' algorithm for deformable image registration in radiation therapy". *Physics in Medicine and Biology*, Vol. 50, No. 12, pp. 1887–2905, June 2005.

[Wang 12]   H. Wang, S. Mossaab, and A. Masood. "Real Time Three-Dimensional Echocardiography in Assessment of Left Ventricular Dyssynchrony and Cardiac Resynchronization Therapy". *Echocardiography*, Vol. 29, No. 2, pp. 192–199, February 2012.

[Wang 13a]   J. Wang and X. Gu. "Simultaneous motion estimation and image reconstruction (SMEIR) for 4D cone-beam CT". *Medical Physics*, Vol. 40, No. 10, pp. 101912-1–11, October 2013.

[Wang 13b]   J. Wang, C. Riess, A. Borsdorf, B. Heigl, and J. Hornegger. "Sparse Depth Sampling for Interventional 2-D/3-D Overlay: Theoretical Error Analysis and Enhanced Motion Estimation". In: R. Wilson, E. Hancock, A. Bors, and W. Smith, Eds., *15th International Conference on Computer Analysis of Images and Patterns 2013*. Springer Verlag Berlin Heidelberg, *August 27-29, 2013, York, UK*. pp. 86–93.

[Wang 13c]   P. Wang, O. Ecabert, T. Chen, M. Wels, J. Rieber, M. Ostermeier, and D. Comaniciu. "Image-based Co-Registration of Angiography and Intravascular Ultrasound Images". *IEEE Transactions on Medical Imaging*, Vol. 32, No. 12, pp. 2238–2249, December 2013.

[Wein 08]   A. Weinlich, B. Keck, H. Scherl, M. Kowarschik, and J. Hornegger. "Comparison of High-Speed Ray Casting on GPU using CUDA and OpenGL". In: R. Buchty and J.-P. Weiß, Eds., *Proceedings of the First International Workshop on New Frontiers in High-performance and Hardware-aware Computing (HipHaC'08)*. Universitätsverlag Karlsruhe, *November 8, 2008, Lake Como, Italy*.

[Wick 13]   J. Wicklein, Y. Kyriakou, W. A. Kalender, and H. Kunze. "An online motion- and misalignment-correction method for medical flat-detector CT". In: R. Nishikawa and B. Whiting, Eds., *Proceedings of SPIE Medical Imaging 2013. February 9-14, 2013, Lake Buena Vista, FL, USA*. p. 86681S.

[Wiel 14]   J.-Y. Wielandts, S. De Buck, J. Ector, D. Nuyens, F. Maes, and H. Heidbuchel. "Registration based filtering: an acceptable tool for noise reduction in left ventricular dynamic rotational angiography images?". In: Z. Yaniv and D. Holmes, Eds., *Proceedings of SPIE Medical Imaging 2014: Image-Guided Procedures, Robotic Interventions, and Modeling. February 15-20, 2014, San Diego, CA, USA*. p. 903628.

[Wies 00]   K. Wiesent, K. Barth, N. Navab, P. Durlak, T. Brunner, O. Schuetz, and W. Seissler. "Enhanced 3-D reconstruction algorithm for C-arm systems suitable for interventional procedures". *IEEE Transactions on Medical Imaging*, Vol. 19, No. 5, pp. 391–403, May 2000.

[Wils 98]   P. W. Wilson, R. B. D'Agostino, D. Levy, A. M. Belanger, H. Silbershatz, and W. B. Kannel. "Prediction of coronary heart disease using risk factor categories". *Circulation*, Vol. 97, No. 18, pp. 1837–1847, May 1998.

[Zell 05]   M. Zellerhoff, B. Scholz, T. Brunner, and E.-P. Ruehrnschopf. "Low contrast 3D reconstruction from C-arm data". In: M. Flynn, Ed., *Proceedings of SPIE Medical Imaging 2005: Physics of Medical Imaging. February 12-18, 2005, San Diego, CA, USA*. p. 646.

[Zeng 09]   G. Zeng. *Medical Image Reconstruction- A Conceptual Tutorial*. Springer Verlag Berlin Heidelberg, 1st Ed., 2009.

[Zhan 11]   Z. Zhang, X. Song, and D. J. Sahn. "Cardiac Motion Estimation from 3D Echocardiography with Spatiotemporal Regularization". In: D. Metaxas and L. Axel, Eds., *Functional Imaging and Modeling of the Heart (FIMH) 2011. Springer Verlag Berlin Heidelberg, May 25-27, 2011, New York City, NY, USA*. pp. 350–358.

[Zhen 08]   Y. Zheng, A. Barbu, B. Georgescu, M. Scheuering, and D. Comaniciu. "Four-chamber heart modeling and automatic segmentation for 3D cardiac CT volumes using marginal space learning and steerable features". *IEEE Transactions on Medical Imaging*, Vol. 27, No. 11, pp. 1668–1681, August 2008.

[Zou 04]   K. H. Zou, S. K. Warfield, A. Bharatha, C. M. Tempany, M. R. Kaus, S. J. Haker, W. M. Wells, F. A. Jolesz, and R. Kikinis. "Statistical validation of image segmentation quality based on a spatial overlap index". *Academic Radiology*, Vol. 11, No. 2, pp. 178–189, March 2004.